The Complete Guide to
Anti-Inflammation
How to Eat Smarter and Live Longer

20 HEALTHY SELF-CARE HABITS

BOOST YOUR HEALTH

PREVENT DISEASES

BETTER SELF CARE

INCREASE ENERGY

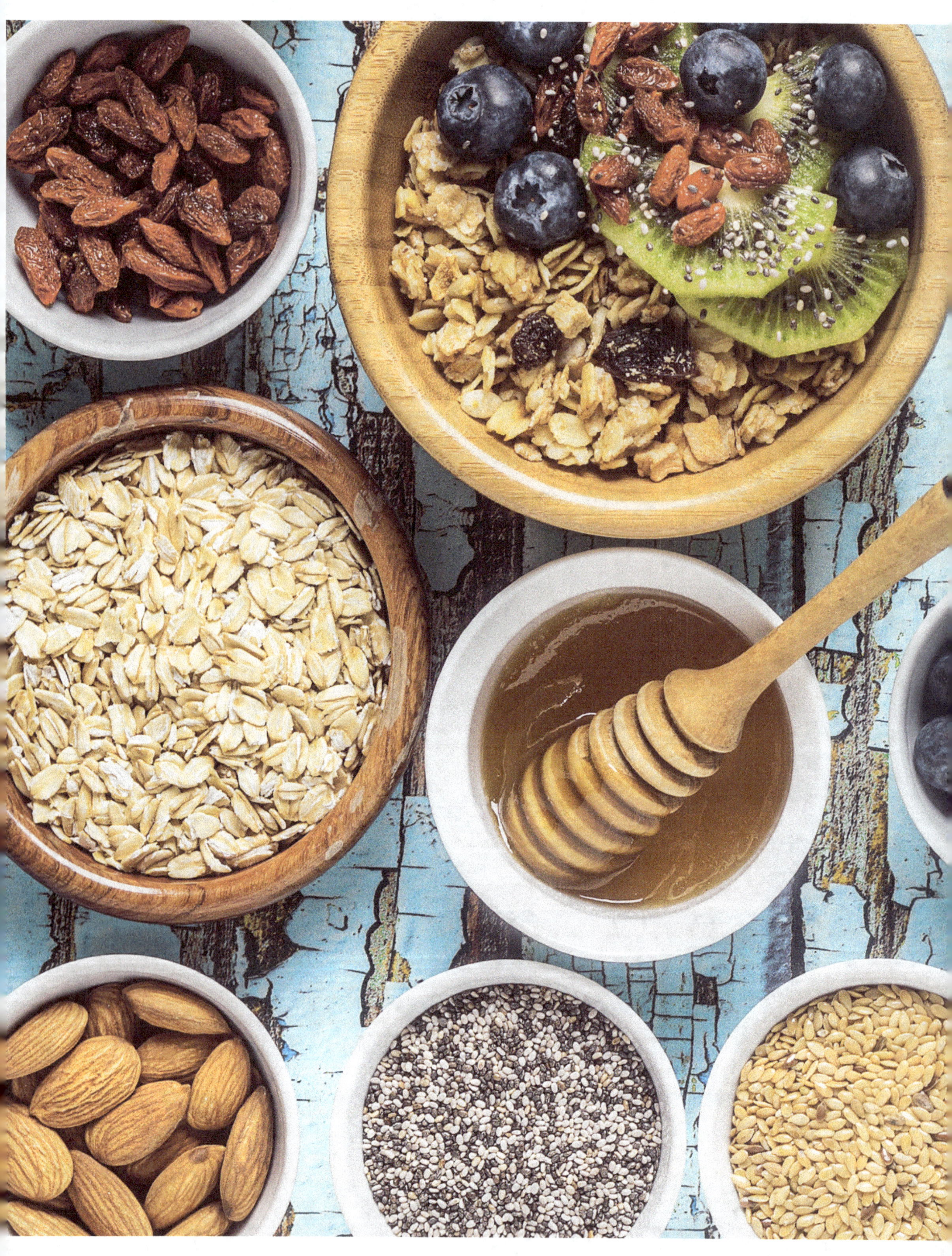

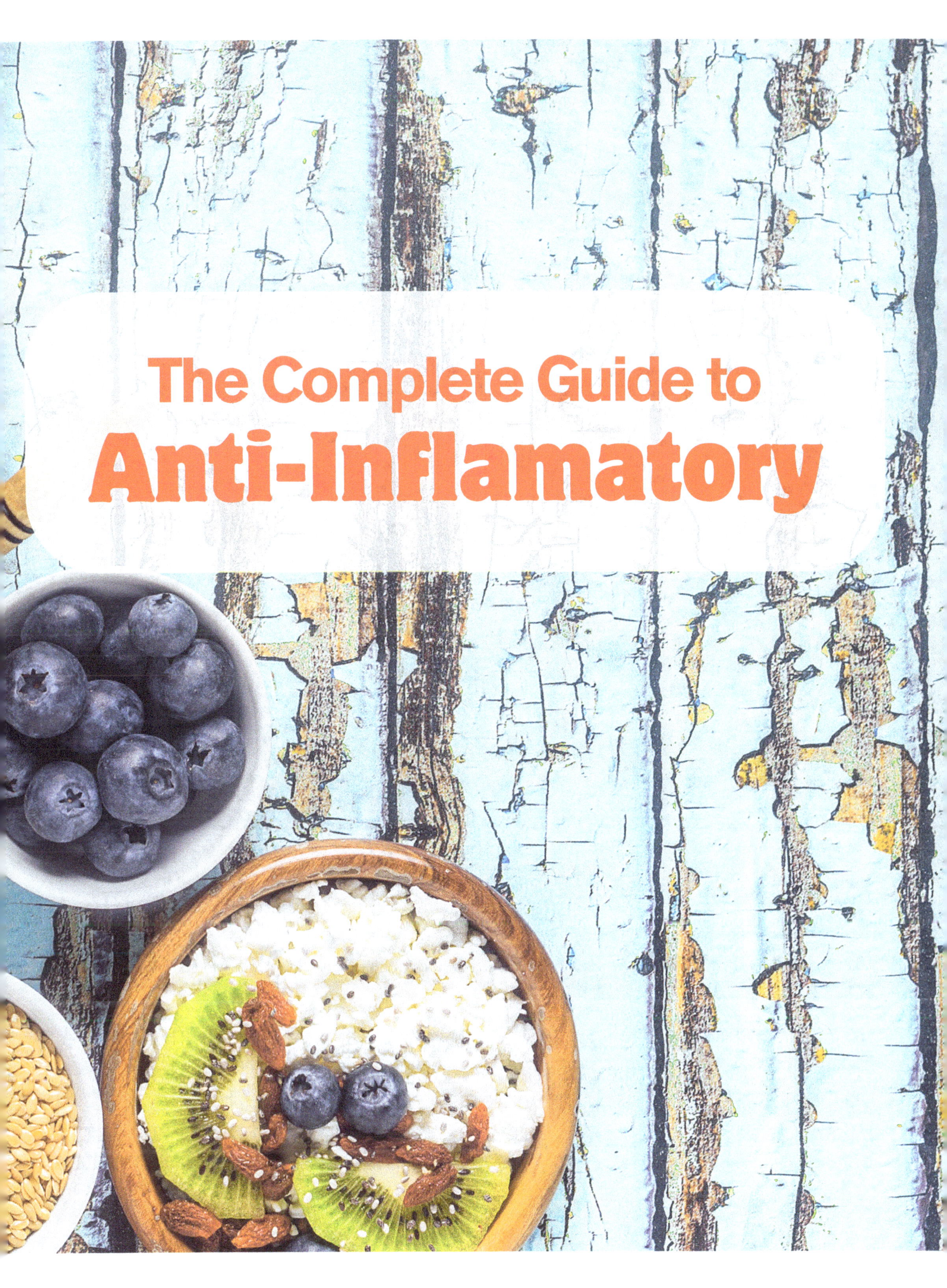

The Complete Guide to
Anti-Inflamatory

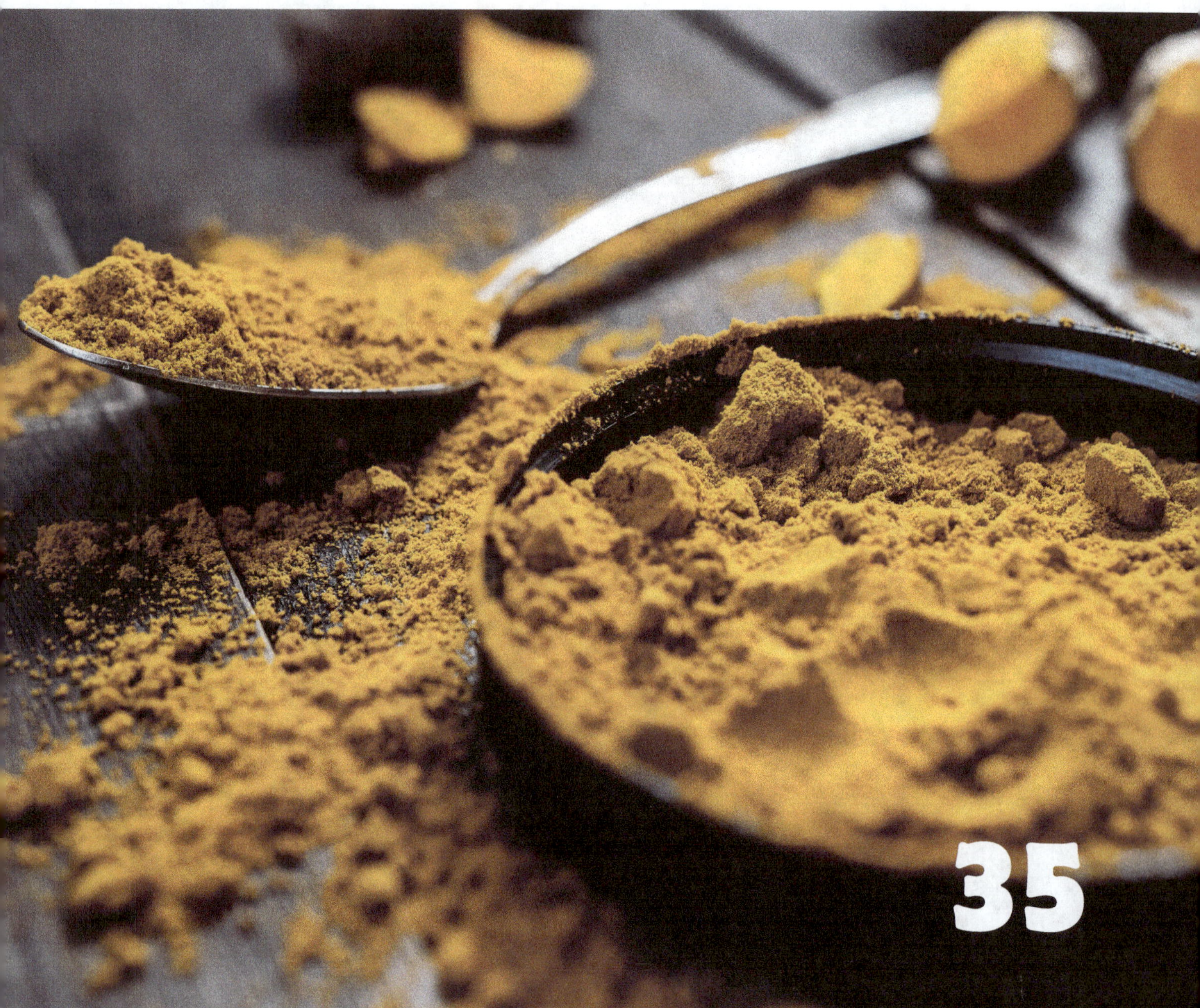

Part 1

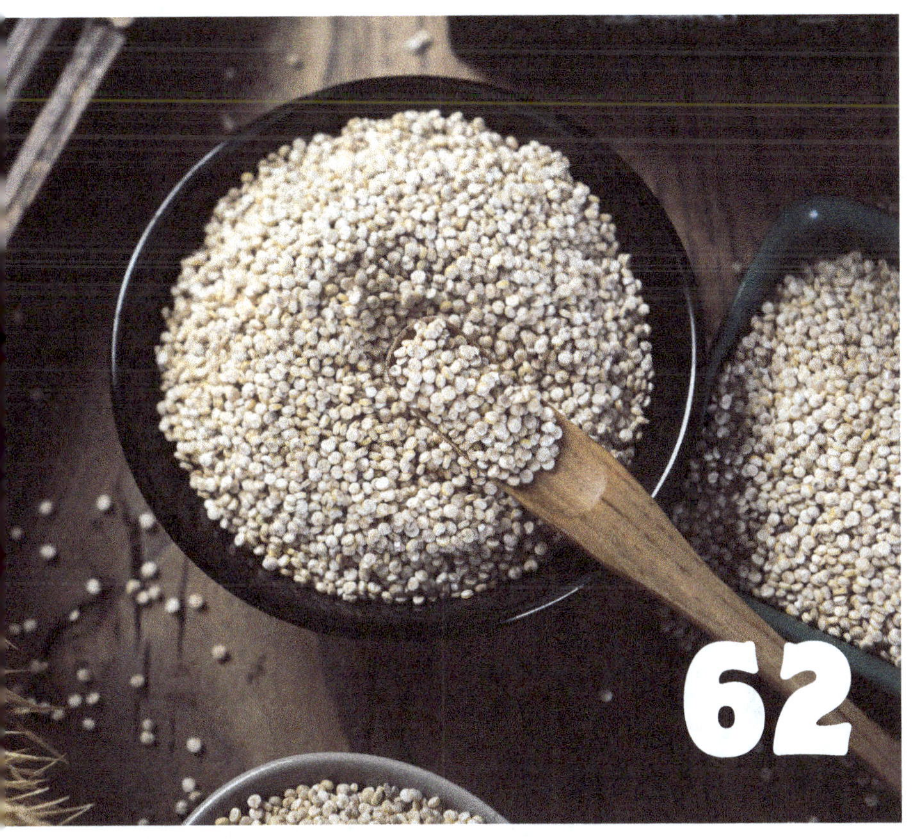

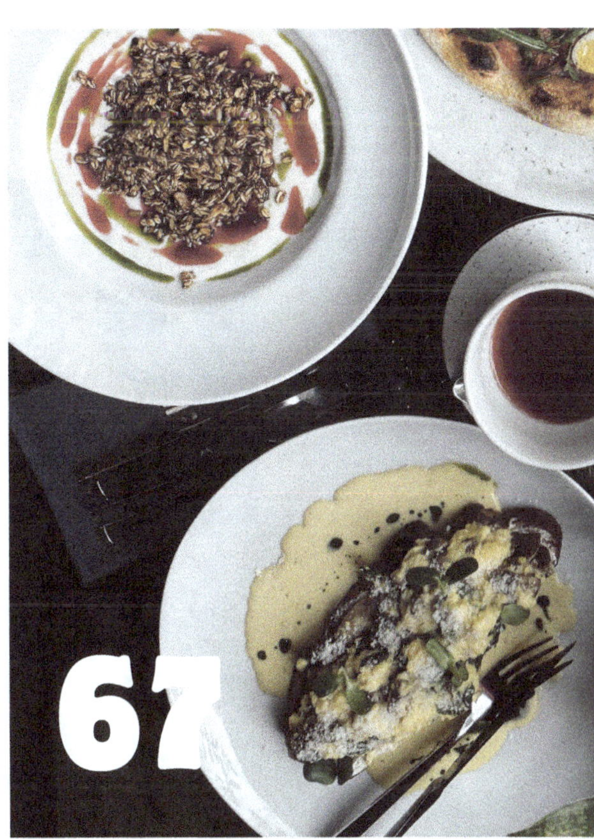

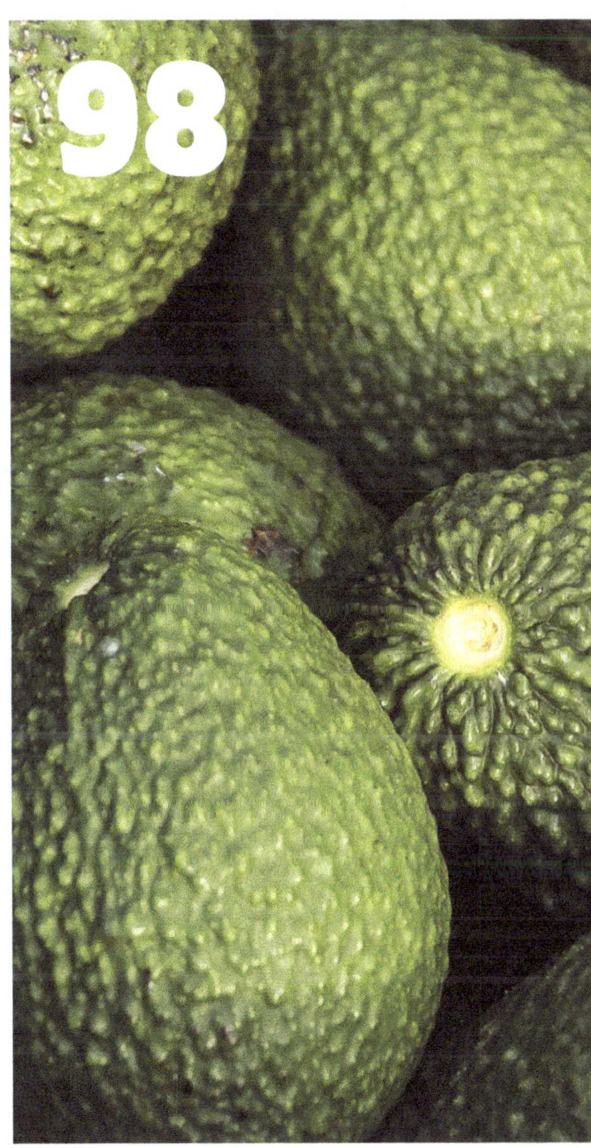

Part 2

60 - Eat Smarter for a Healthier You

PART 1

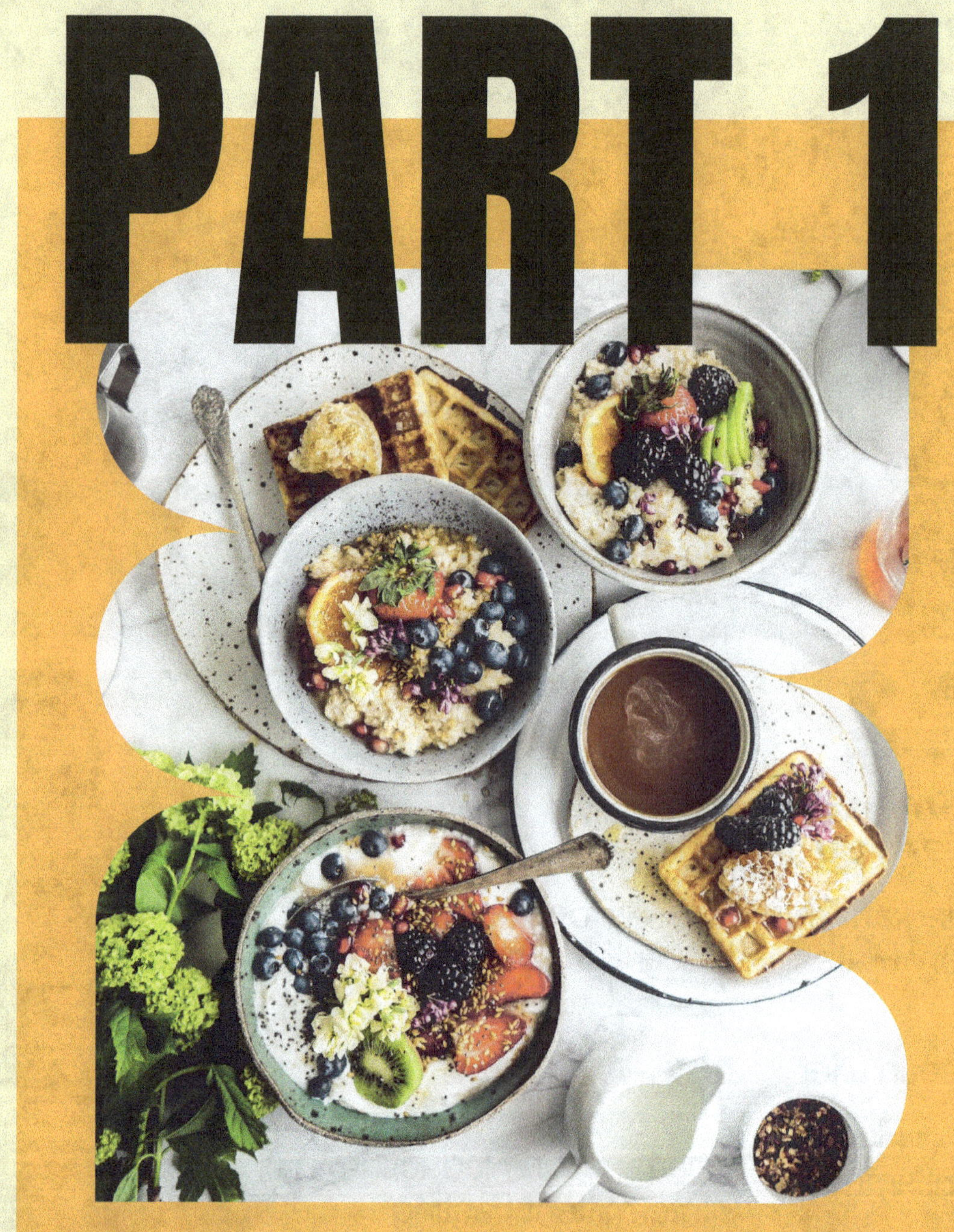

THE ROADMAP TO A HEALTHIER YOU

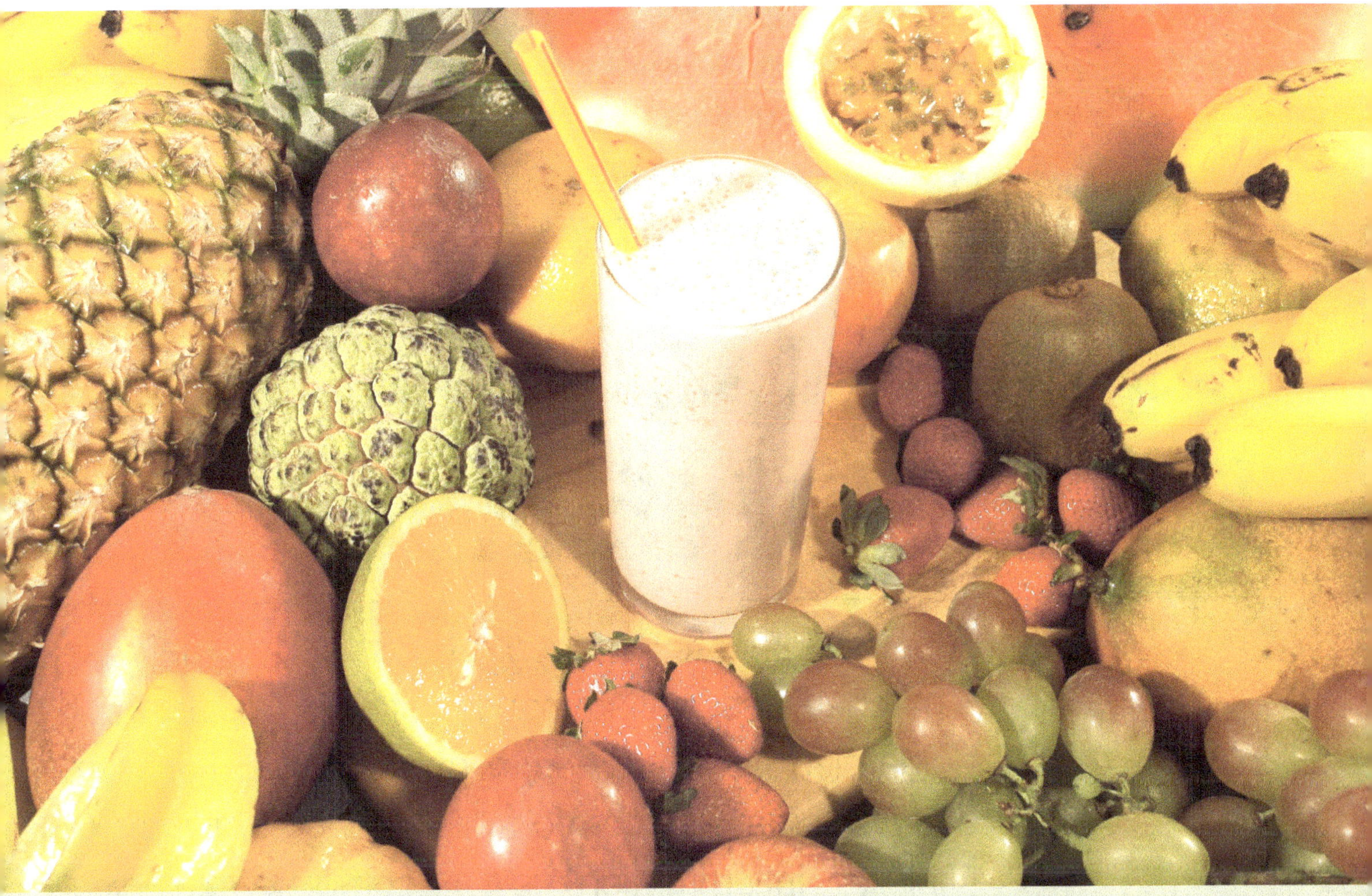

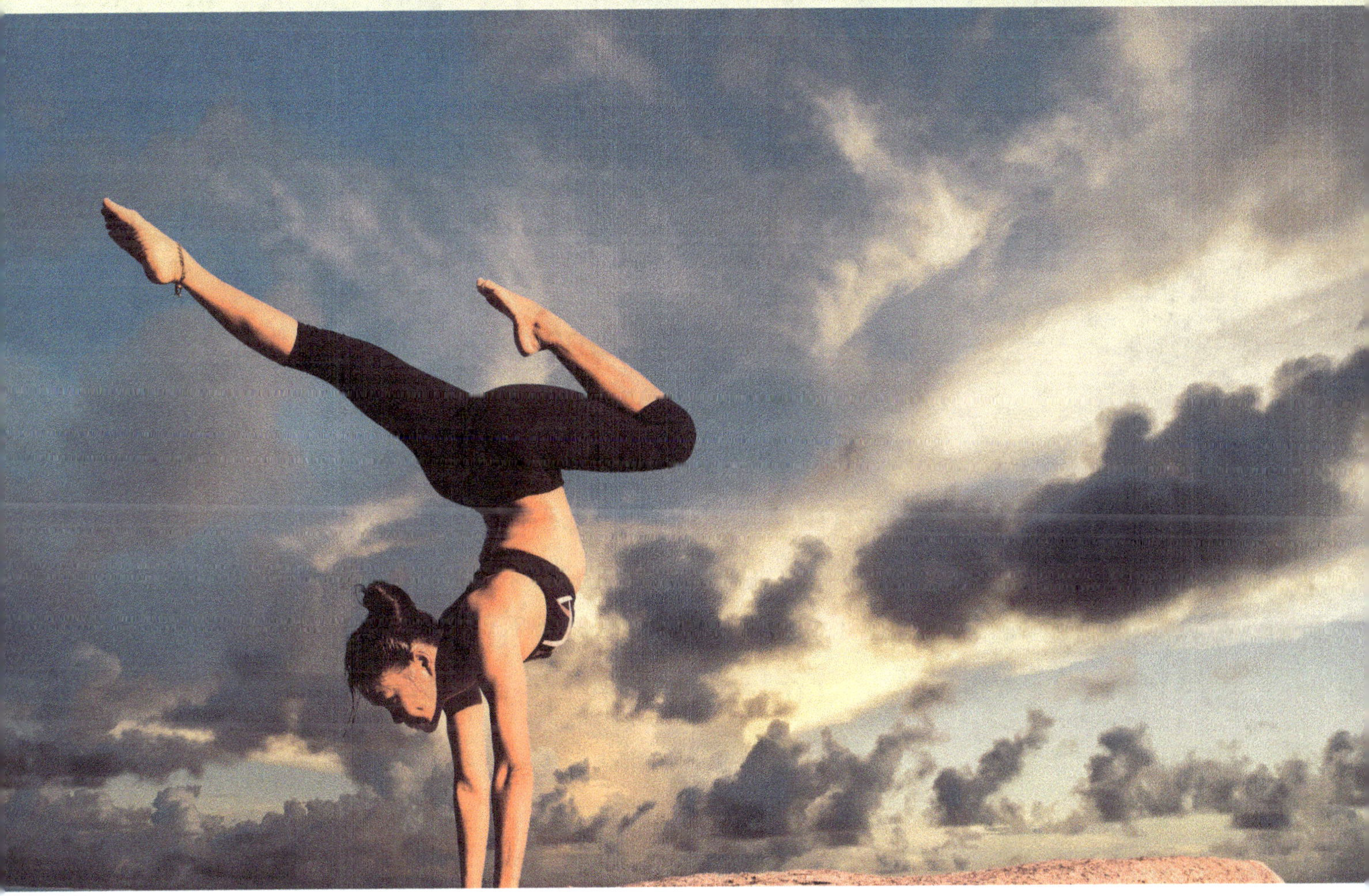

UNDERSTANDING THE BODY'S RESPONSE

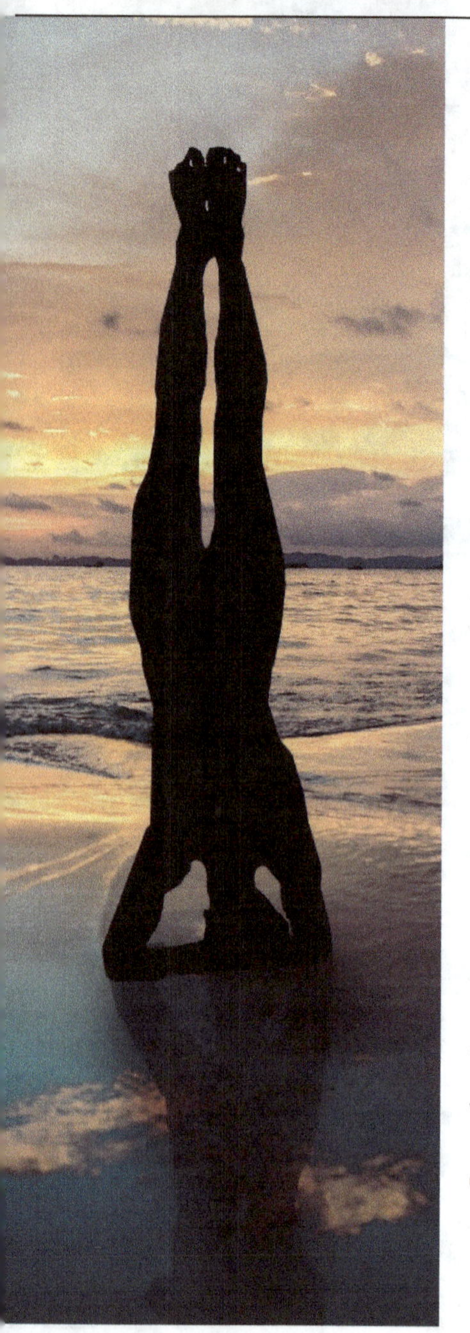

In the intricate tapestry of our body's defense mechanisms, inflammation stands as both a guardian and, at times, a potential foe. Far from being a mere discomfort or swelling after a minor injury, inflammation is a complex biological response that plays a pivotal role in our overall health. To truly embark on a journey toward a healthier, inflammation-free life, we must first unravel the mysteries behind this bodily process.

At its core, inflammation is a natural and necessary response triggered by the immune system. When the body detects injury, infection, or harmful stimuli, a cascade of events is set into motion. Blood vessels dilate, allowing immune cells to rush to the affected area. These cells work tirelessly to neutralize invaders, repair damaged tissues, and restore balance.

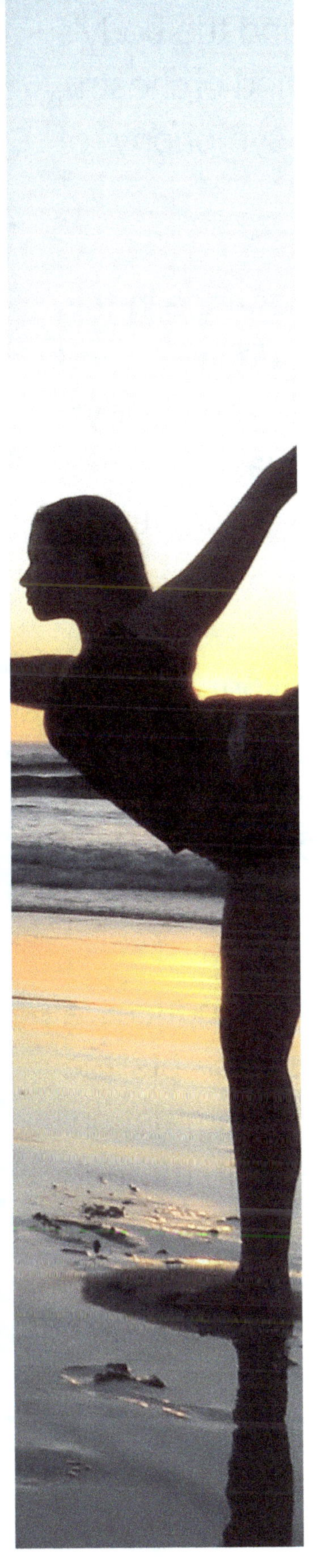

While acute inflammation is a temporary and localized response crucial for healing, chronic inflammation is a more insidious adversary. Prolonged inflammation, often unnoticed, can lead to a range of health issues, including heart disease, diabetes, and autoimmune disorders. Understanding the triggers of chronic inflammation is the first step in taking control of our well-being.

Modern lifestyles, characterized by poor dietary choices, sedentary habits, and chronic stress, contribute significantly to the prevalence of chronic inflammation. Processed foods high in sugars and unhealthy fats, coupled with a lack of exercise, create a perfect storm within our bodies, fueling the flames of persistent inflammation.

Fortunately, knowledge is power. Armed with an understanding of the factors that contribute to inflammation, we can make informed choices to mitigate its effects. In the upcoming articles, we will explore the impact of diet, exercise, stress management, and sleep on inflammation levels. We will delve into the world of anti-inflammatory superfoods and lifestyle changes that promote a balanced, inflammation-resistant body.

As we navigate the terrain of inflammation, it's essential to recognize the profound interconnection between lifestyle choices and the body's inflammatory response. Imagine your body as a finely tuned orchestra, and inflammation as the conductor orchestrating a symphony of healing or, in some cases, discord.

The foods we consume serve as either harmony or dissonance in this symphony. Processed foods laden with artificial additives and excessive sugars can be likened to a cacophony, sending the body's inflammatory markers into overdrive. Conversely, embracing a diet rich in whole, nutrient-dense foods becomes the melody, promoting a harmonious balance within.

Exercise, too, plays a key role in this intricate composition. Physical activity not only keeps the body agile but also acts as a soothing balm for inflammation. Engaging in regular exercise helps regulate the immune system, keeping inflammation in check and promoting overall well-being.

Stress, a ubiquitous companion in our fast-paced lives, introduces a discordant note to the melody of health. Chronic stress prompts the release of stress hormones, perpetuating a state of inflammation. However, adopting stress management techniques—be it through meditation, deep breathing, or mindfulness—can harmonize the body's response, fostering a calm and balanced internal environment.

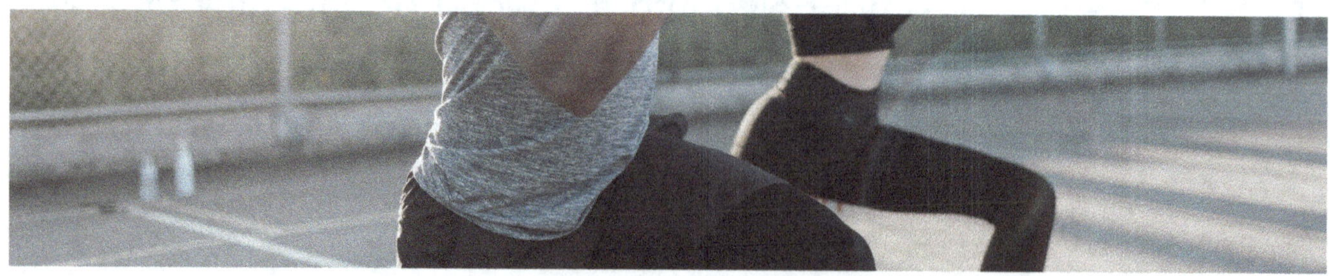

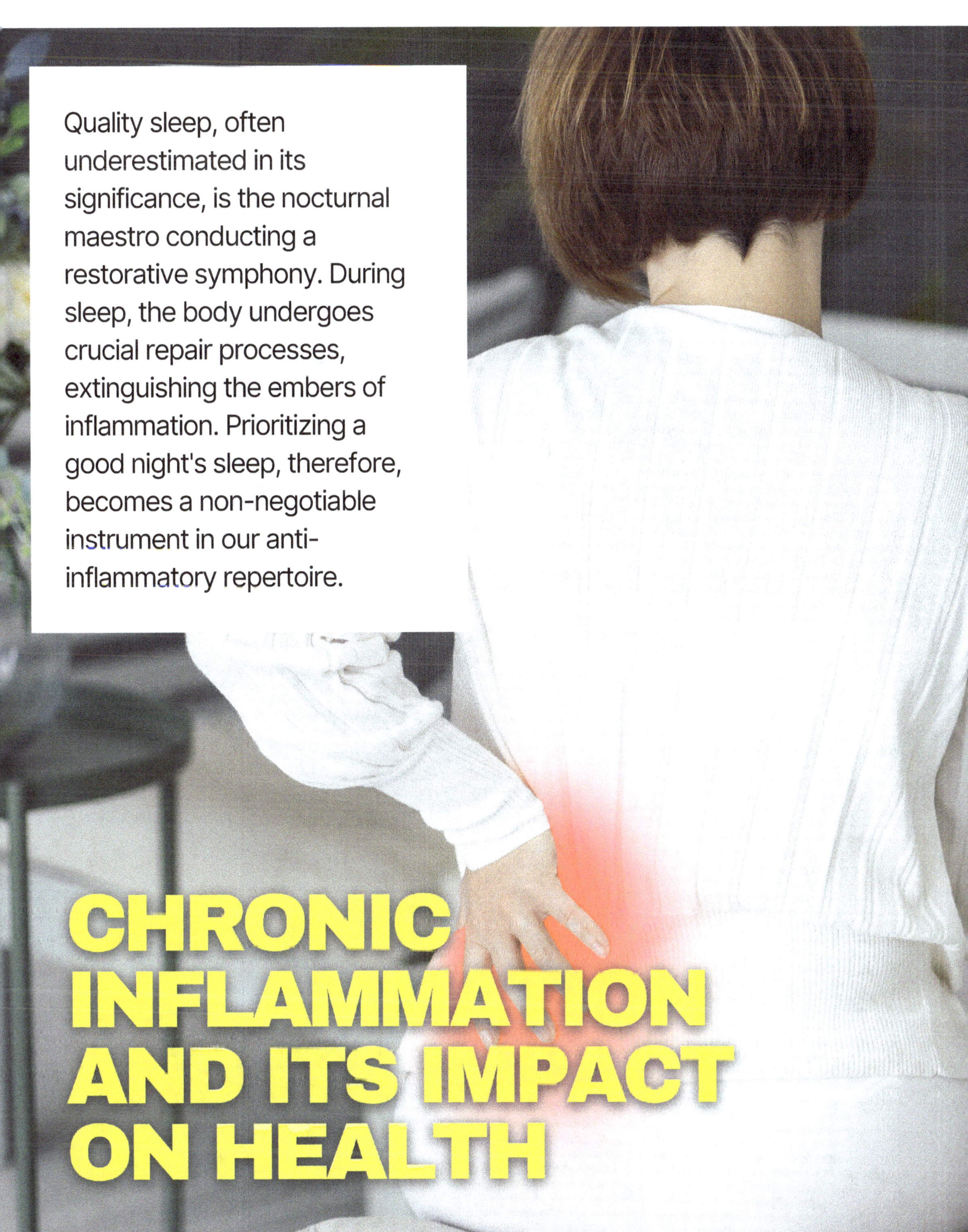

Quality sleep, often underestimated in its significance, is the nocturnal maestro conducting a restorative symphony. During sleep, the body undergoes crucial repair processes, extinguishing the embers of inflammation. Prioritizing a good night's sleep, therefore, becomes a non-negotiable instrument in our anti-inflammatory repertoire.

CHRONIC INFLAMMATION AND ITS IMPACT ON HEALTH

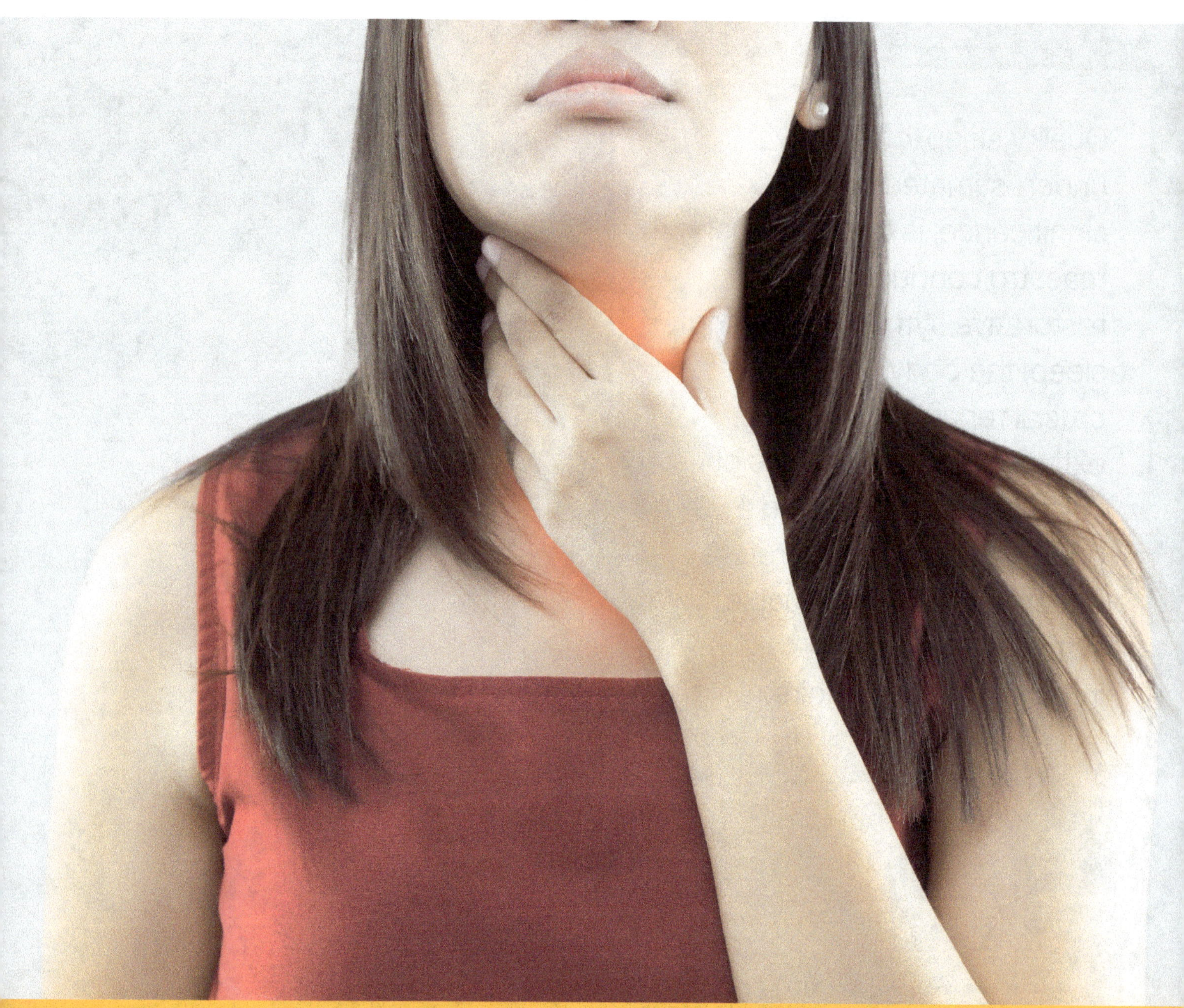

CHRONIC INFLAMMATION AND ITS IMPACT ON HEALTH

In the intricate dance of our body's defense mechanisms, inflammation is a natural response to injury or infection. It's the cavalry rushing to the rescue, signaling the immune system to heal and protect. However, when inflammation becomes chronic, it transforms from a helpful ally into a silent and destructive foe, wreaking havoc on our health in ways we may not immediately recognize.

Chronic inflammation is like a smoldering fire beneath the surface, persisting over the long term. Unlike acute inflammation, which is a rapid and temporary response to an injury or infection, chronic inflammation is subtle, often unnoticed until it begins to manifest in various health issues. This low-grade inflammation can be triggered by factors such as poor diet, stress, lack of exercise, and environmental toxins.

The consequences of chronic inflammation are far-reaching, affecting nearly every system in the body. One of its primary dangers lies in its ability to contribute to the development of various chronic diseases. Heart disease, diabetes, arthritis, and even certain types of cancer have been linked to prolonged inflammation. It's like a domino effect, with the inflammatory response disrupting the delicate balance required for optimal health.

The cardiovascular system is particularly vulnerable to the effects of chronic inflammation. Prolonged inflammation can damage blood vessels and contribute to the buildup of arterial plaque, increasing the risk of heart attacks and strokes. Additionally, chronic inflammation may exacerbate existing heart conditions, creating a dangerous cycle that compromises cardiovascular health.

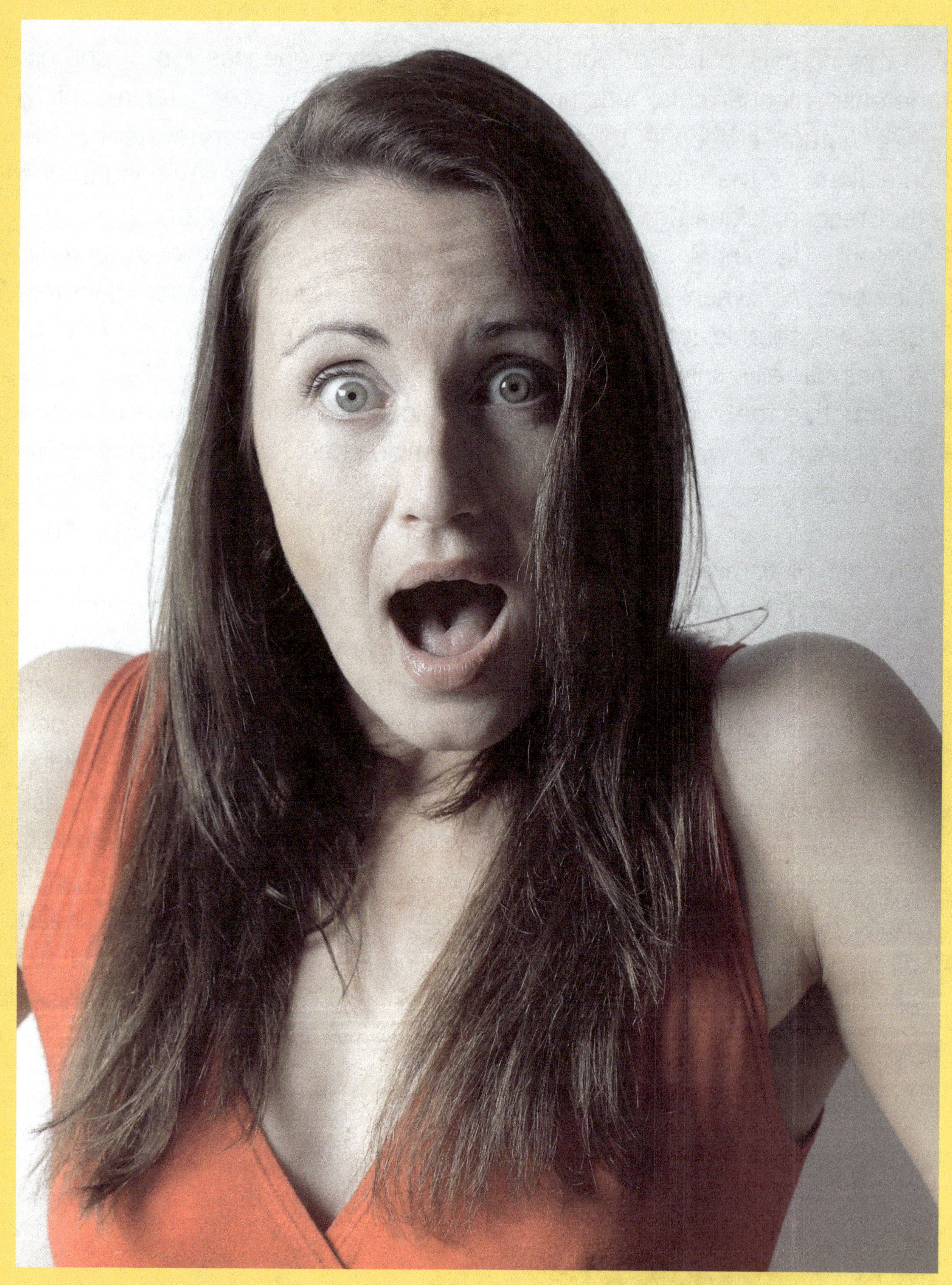

Inflammatory Links to Metabolic Disorders

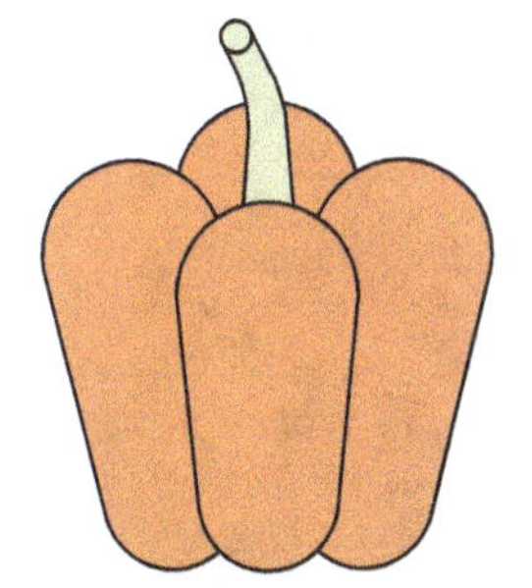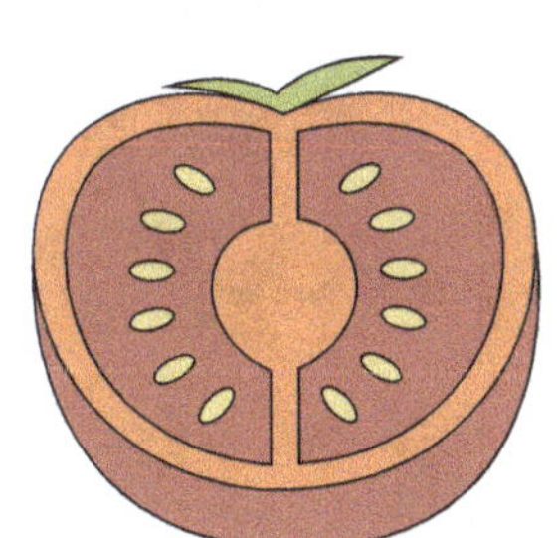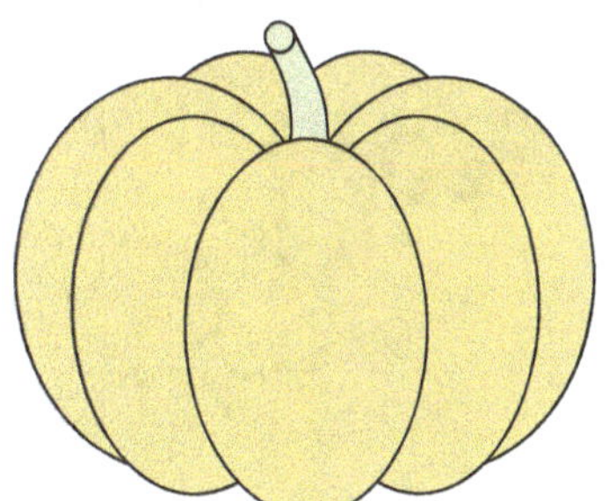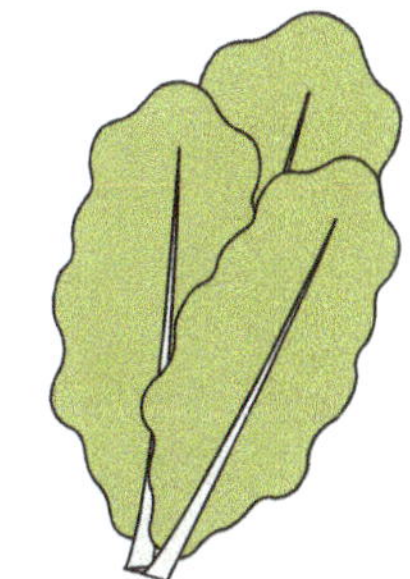

Chronic inflammation plays a pivotal role in metabolic disorders such as diabetes and obesity.

Insulin resistance, a key factor in type 2 diabetes, can be exacerbated by inflammatory processes. Adipose tissue, commonly known as fat cells, produces inflammatory substances, further contributing to the chronic inflammation associated with obesity.

Inflammation and joint pain often go hand in hand, as seen in conditions like rheumatoid arthritis. Chronic inflammation can lead to the destruction of joint tissues, causing pain, stiffness, and reduced mobility. Understanding and managing inflammation is crucial for those dealing with chronic joint conditions.

In recent years, there has been a growing understanding of the connection between chronic inflammation and neurological disorders like Alzheimer's and Parkinson's disease. The impact of inflammation in the brain is increasingly recognized as a factor that may contribute to the progression of these conditions. This emphasizes the importance of addressing inflammation not only for physical health but also for cognitive well-being.

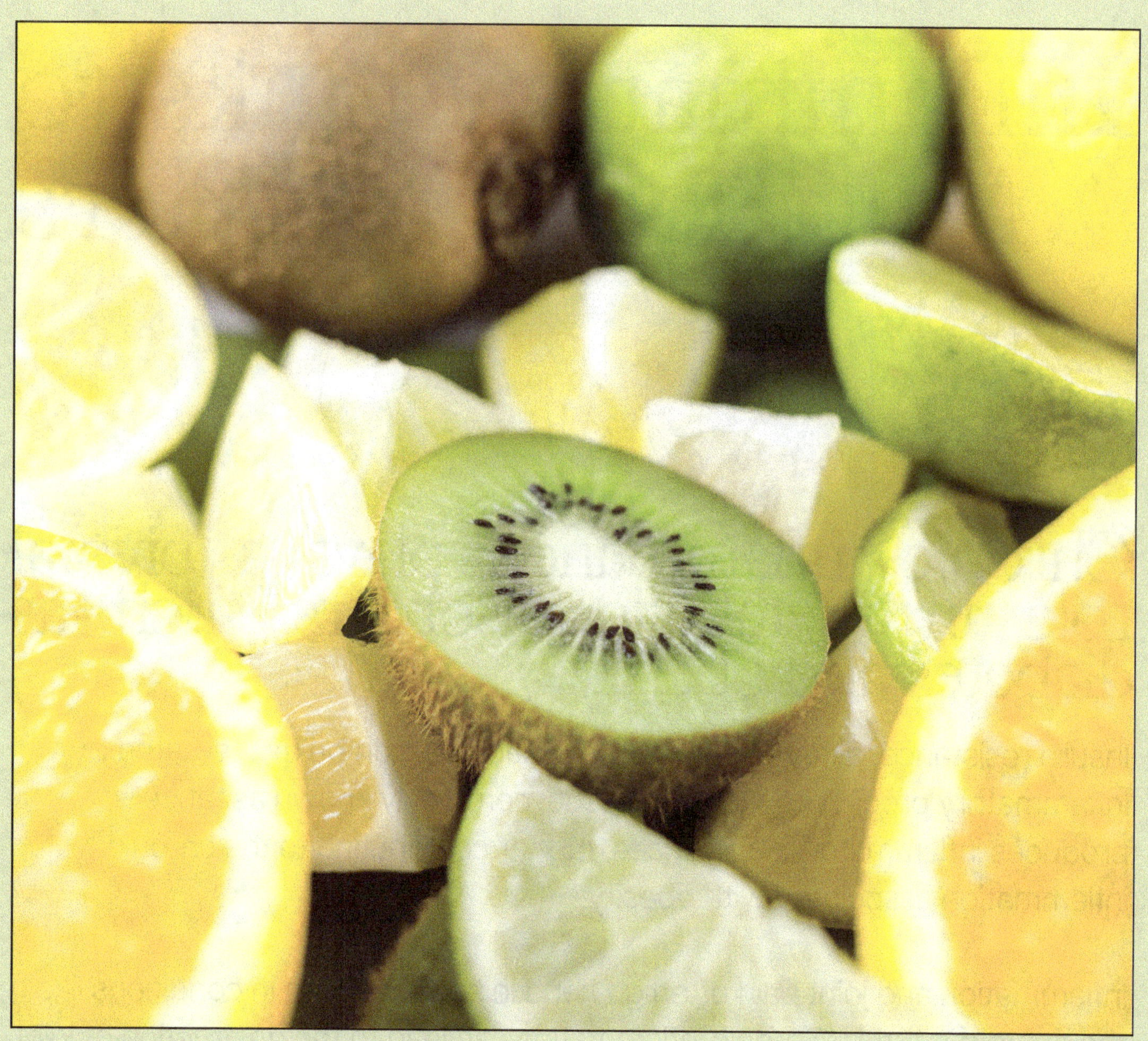

The good news is that lifestyle choices can significantly impact the level of inflammation in the body. Adopting an anti-inflammatory diet rich in fruits, vegetables, and omega-3 fatty acids, along with regular exercise and stress management, can help keep chronic inflammation in check.

As we unravel the complexities of chronic inflammation, it becomes clear that this silent assailant requires our attention. Acknowledging the connection between inflammation and overall health empowers us to make informed choices, paving the way for a life of vitality and well-being. By understanding and addressing chronic inflammation, we take a proactive step toward a healthier and more resilient future.

INFLAMMATORY FOODS TO AVOID

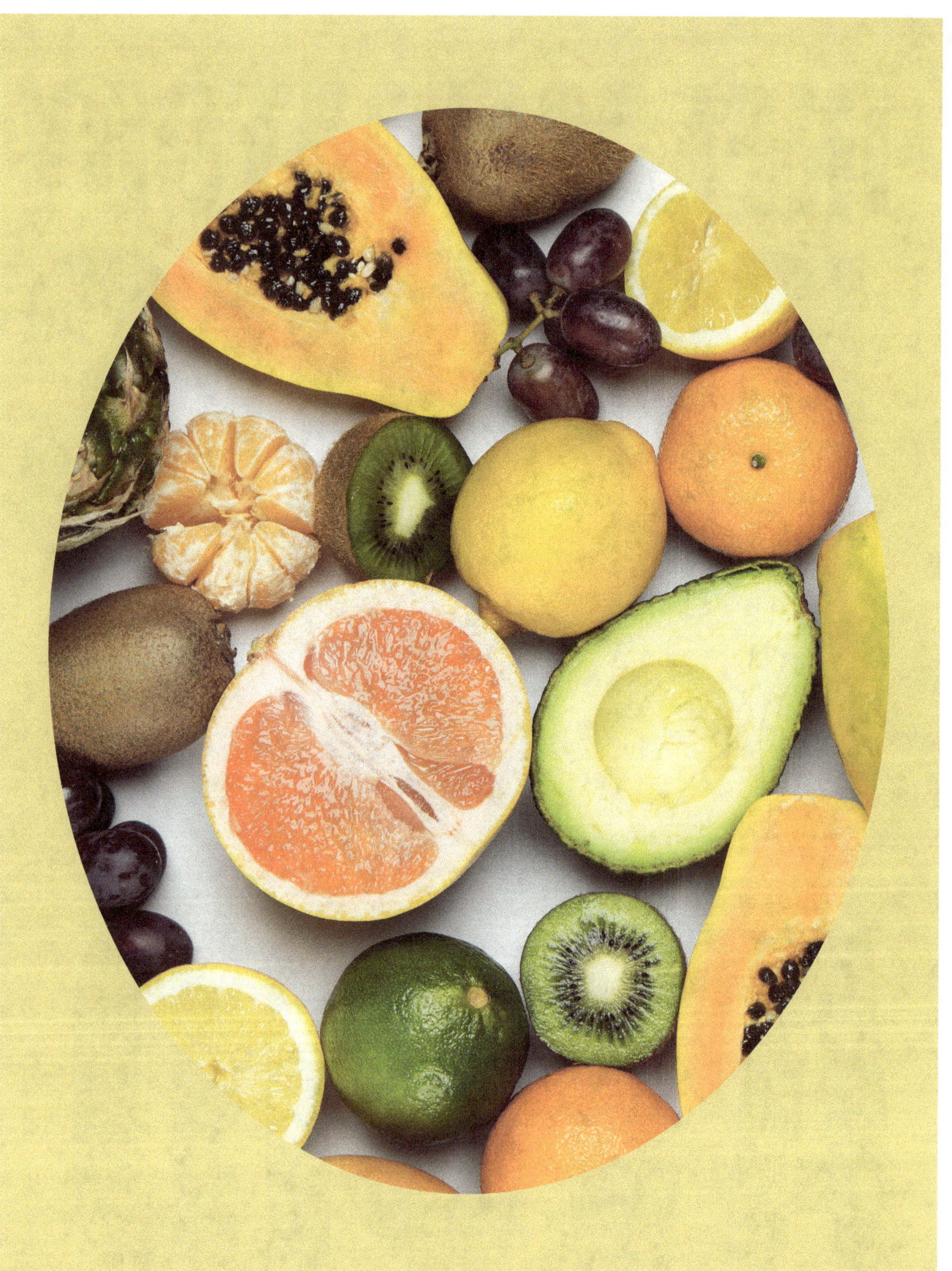

In the pursuit of optimal health, the role of our diet cannot be overstated. What we choose to put on our plates can either fuel our bodies with vitality or contribute to a state of chronic inflammation, a precursor to various health issues. Let's embark on a journey of dietary awareness as we explore the inflammatory foods that might be silently sabotaging our well-being.

Refined Sugars and Artificial Sweeteners
The sweet satisfaction from indulging in sugary treats often comes at a cost. Refined sugars, prevalent in candies, sodas, and processed snacks, are known to trigger inflammation. Likewise, artificial sweeteners, though marketed as sugar substitutes, may disrupt the balance of gut bacteria, contributing to an inflammatory response.

Processed and Red Meats
Processed meats, such as sausages and hot dogs, are not only linked to cardiovascular issues but also to inflammation. Similarly, red meats, especially those high in saturated fats, can promote inflammation in the body. Opting for lean protein sources like poultry, fish, or plant-based alternatives can be a wiser choice.

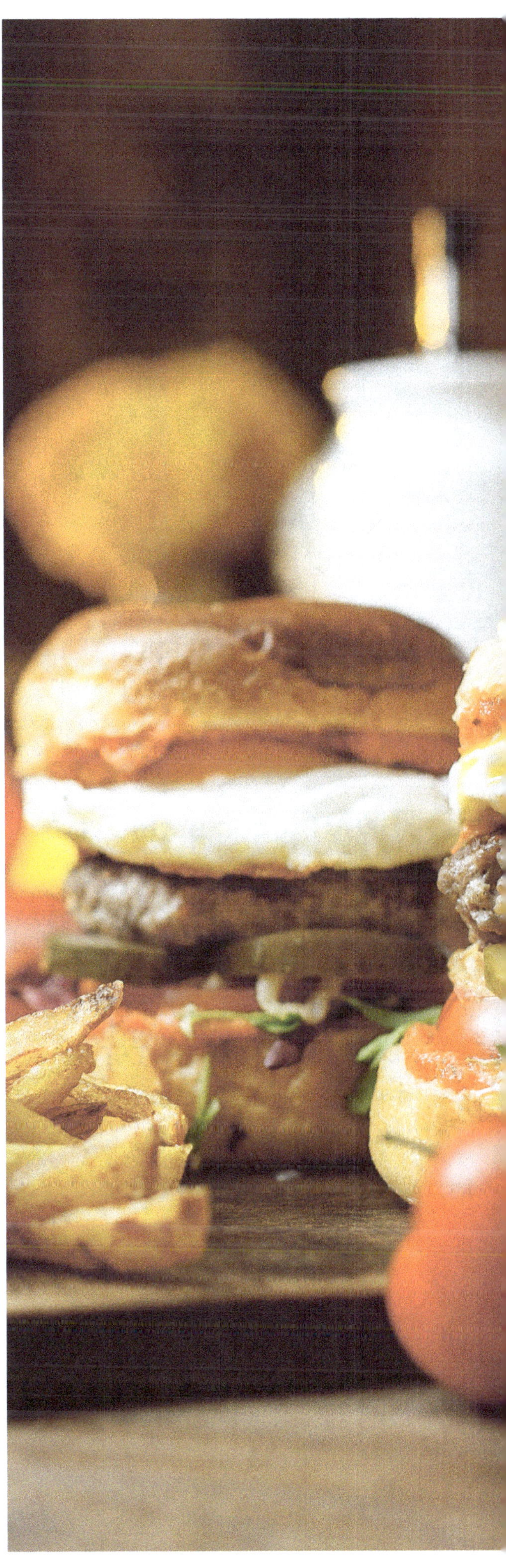

Highly Processed Foods and Additives

The convenience of highly processed foods often comes with a hidden cost. These items are frequently loaded with additives, preservatives, and unhealthy fats, all of which can trigger inflammation. Opting for whole, unprocessed foods and cooking from scratch empowers you to control what goes into your meals.

Dairy Products with A1 Casein

Some individuals may find that dairy products containing A1 casein, a type of protein found in certain cow's milk, can contribute to inflammation and digestive issues. Exploring alternative dairy options like those made from goat's milk or plant-based alternatives might be a suitable choice for those sensitive to A1 casein.

Excessive Omega-6 Fatty Acids

While omega-6 fatty acids are essential for the body, an imbalance between omega-6 and omega-3 fatty acids can contribute to inflammation. Limiting the intake of vegetable oils like corn, soybean, and sunflower oil, which are high in omega-6, and incorporating more omega-3-rich foods like fatty fish, flaxseeds, and walnuts can help restore balance.

Nightshade Vegetables for Some Individuals

While vegetables are generally considered healthy, some people may experience inflammatory responses to nightshade vegetables like tomatoes, peppers, and eggplants. Observing how your body reacts to these vegetables can help identify any potential sensitivity.

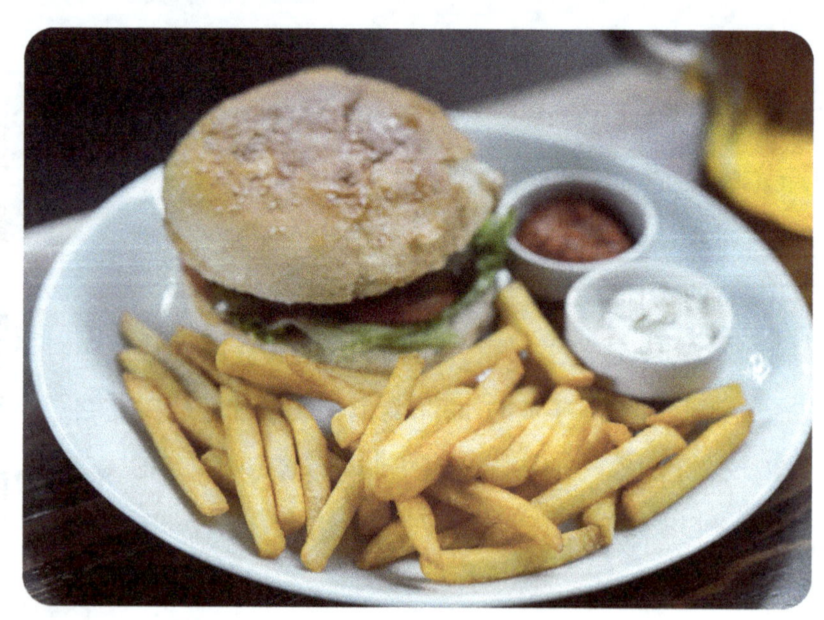

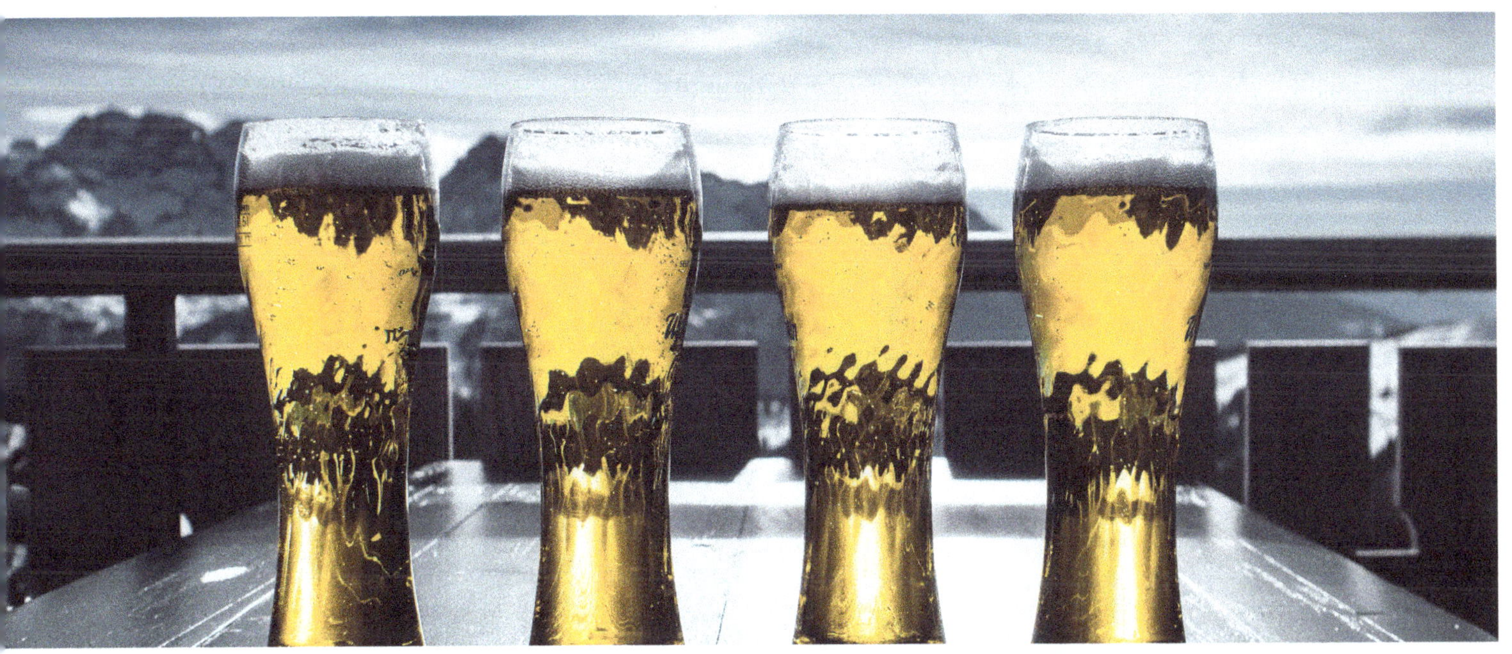

ALCOHOL
in Excess

While moderate alcohol consumption may have certain health benefits, excessive intake can lead to inflammation and negatively impact various organs, particularly the liver. Practicing moderation and being mindful of alcohol consumption contributes to overall well-being.

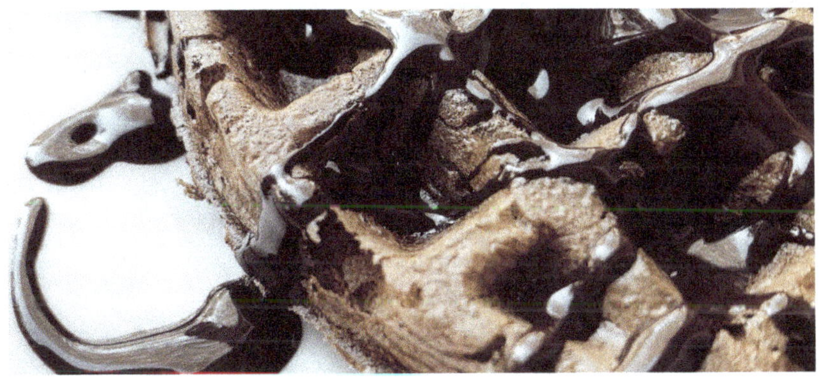

Artificial Additives and High Fructose Corn Syrup

Artificial additives and high fructose corn syrup, commonly found in processed foods and sugary beverages, can contribute to inflammation. Reading labels and opting for natural, whole food alternatives minimizes exposure to these potentially harmful substances.

In the journey toward a healthier lifestyle, being mindful of the foods we consume plays a pivotal role. By steering clear of inflammatory foods and embracing a diet rich in whole, nutrient-dense options, we pave the way for a life marked by vitality and longevity. Your plate is not just a source of nourishment; it's a powerful tool in your quest for optimal well-being.

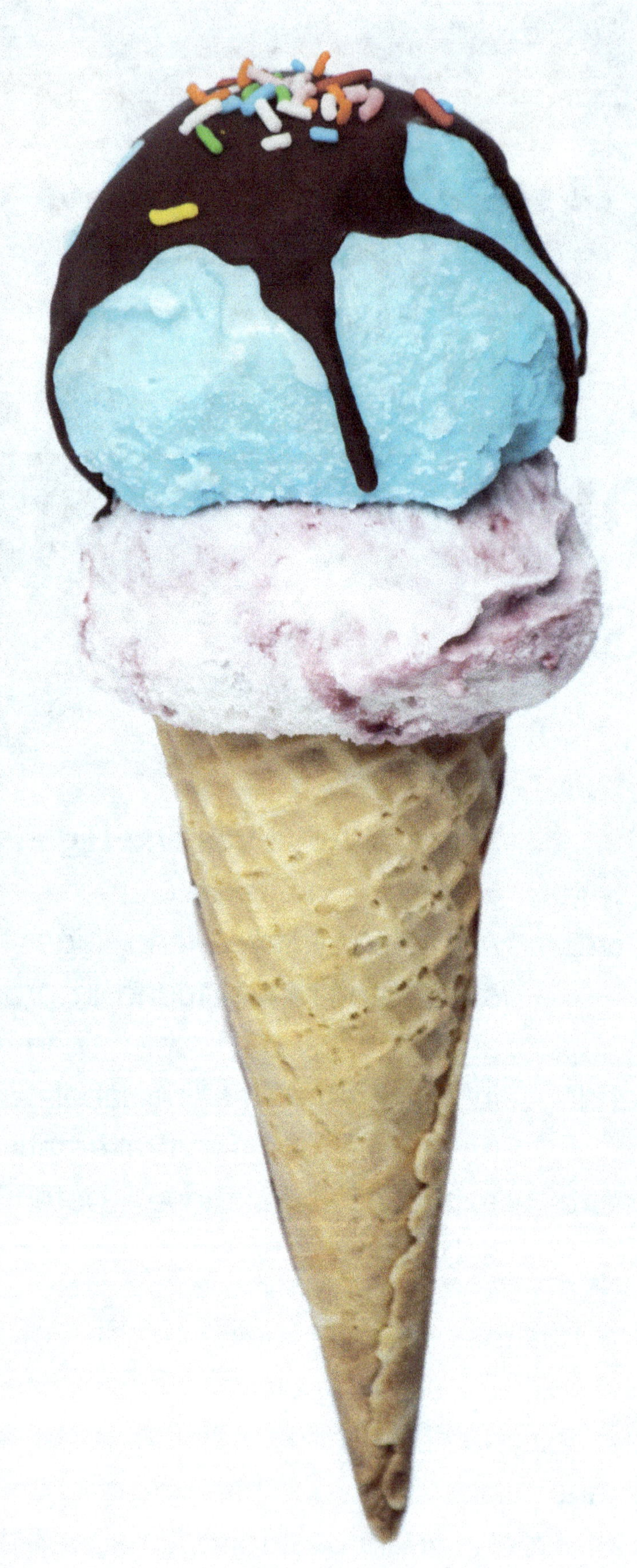

EXERCISE AND INFLAMMATION

IN THE SYMPHONY OF HEALTH, EXERCISE EMERGES AS A POWERFUL CONDUCTOR, ORCHESTRATING A MYRIAD OF PHYSIOLOGICAL RESPONSES THAT EXTEND FAR BEYOND THE REALMS OF WEIGHT MANAGEMENT AND MUSCLE TONE.

One of the fascinating chapters in this intricate story is the relationship between exercise and inflammation. Contrary to a common misconception that exercise may exacerbate inflammation, scientific evidence underscores the profound anti-inflammatory effects of regular physical activity. Let's delve into the dynamic interplay between exercise and inflammation, unraveling the mechanisms that make them a formidable duo in the pursuit of optimal health.

The Paradox of Exercise-Induced Inflammation

Exercise induces a transient inflammatory response in the body, particularly during intense or prolonged bouts of physical activity. This process involves the release of cytokines, small proteins that play a key role in cell signaling and inflammation. While this may sound counterintuitive, this acute, short-term inflammation is a crucial part of the body's adaptation to exercise stress. It serves as a signal to initiate repair and remodeling processes, allowing the body to become more resilient and efficient in handling future challenges.

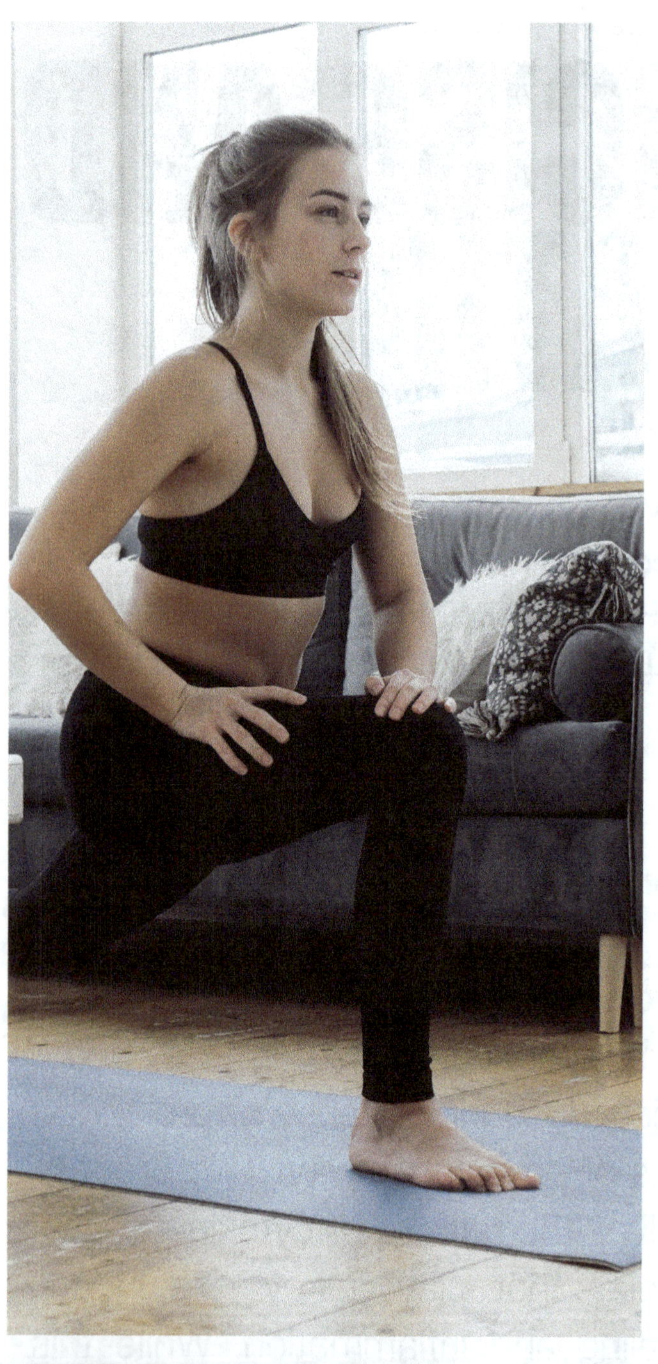

The Anti-Inflammatory Effects of Regular Exercise

The magic unfolds in the aftermath of acute exercise-induced inflammation. As the body adapts to the stress of physical activity, it becomes more adept at managing inflammation, leading to a state of chronic, low-grade inflammation reduction. Regular exercise promotes a balanced immune response, enhancing the body's ability to regulate inflammation and improving overall immune function.

Impact on Systemic Inflammation

Exercise doesn't just confine its anti-inflammatory effects to the muscles; it extends its influence systemically. Studies have consistently shown that individuals who engage in regular, moderate-intensity exercise exhibit lower levels of systemic inflammation markers. This reduction in inflammation contributes to the protective effects of exercise against chronic diseases.

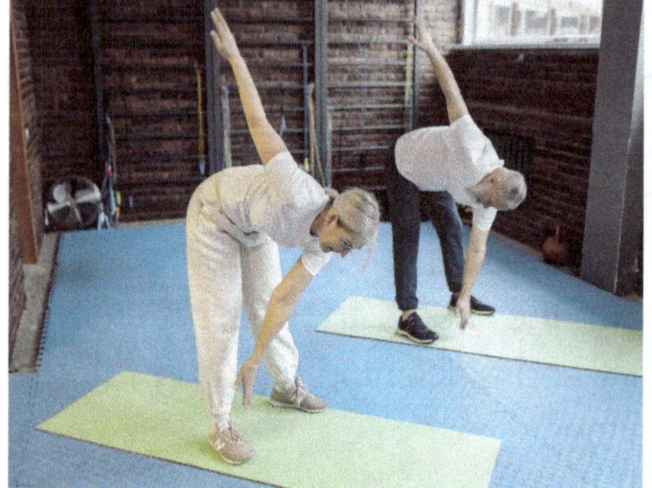

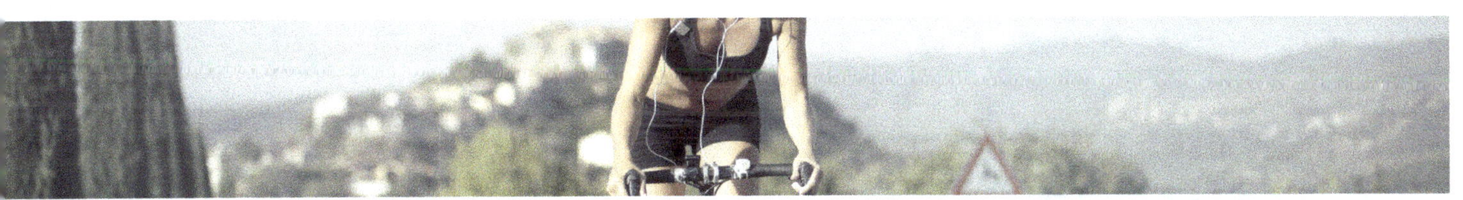

Exercise as a Modulator of Adipose Tissue Inflammation

Adipose tissue, commonly known as fat, is not merely a passive reservoir for energy storage. It's an active endocrine organ that releases signaling molecules, including inflammatory cytokines. Regular exercise has been demonstrated to modulate the inflammatory environment within adipose tissue, promoting a healthier balance of adipokines that positively influence metabolism and inflammation regulation.

The Role of Intensity and Duration

The anti-inflammatory effects of exercise are influenced by factors such as the intensity and duration of physical activity. While moderate-intensity exercise is generally associated with anti-inflammatory benefits, extreme or prolonged exercise, such as marathon running, may temporarily elevate inflammation markers. Striking the right balance is essential, emphasizing the importance of incorporating varied exercise modalities into a well-rounded fitness routine.

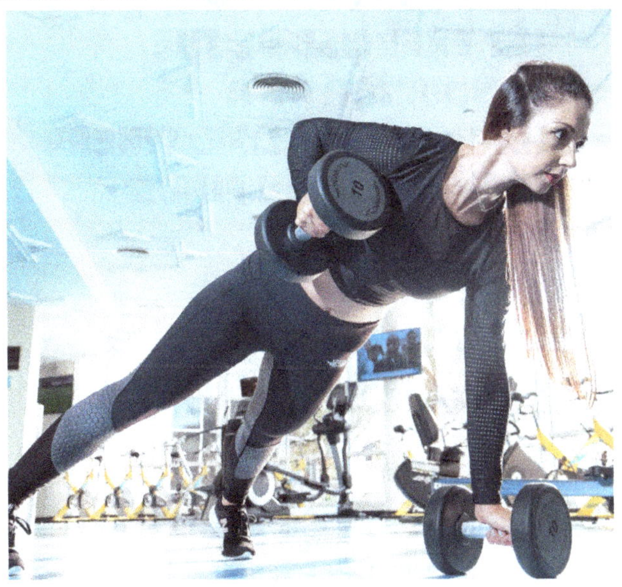

Choosing the Right Exercise Prescription

Different forms of exercise may exert distinct effects on inflammation. Both aerobic exercise, such as jogging or swimming, and resistance training, like weightlifting, contribute to the anti-inflammatory milieu. Finding a personalized exercise routine that combines aerobic and resistance training based on individual preferences and health goals can optimize the anti-inflammatory benefits.

Incorporating Exercise into a Holistic Wellness Strategy

While exercise plays a pivotal role in managing inflammation, its effects are most potent when integrated into a holistic approach to wellness. A balanced and nutrient-dense diet, sufficient sleep, stress management, and regular physical activity collectively create a synergistic environment that fosters overall health and resilience.

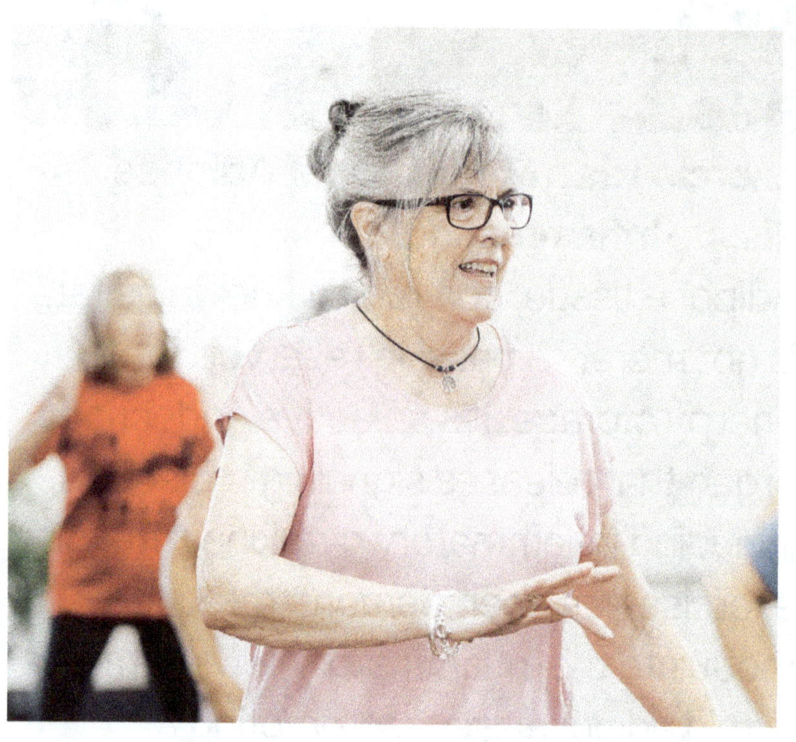

In the intricate dance between exercise and inflammation, the verdict is clear—regular physical activity is a formidable ally in the quest for optimal health. Far from fueling chronic inflammation, exercise emerges as a regulator, fine-tuning the body's inflammatory response for enhanced well-being. Embracing a lifestyle that incorporates varied and enjoyable forms of exercise sets the stage for a life marked by vitality, resilience, and a reduced risk of chronic diseases. The journey toward optimal health is not a sprint but a marathon, and with every step, the dynamic duo of exercise and inflammation propels us forward on this exhilarating path.

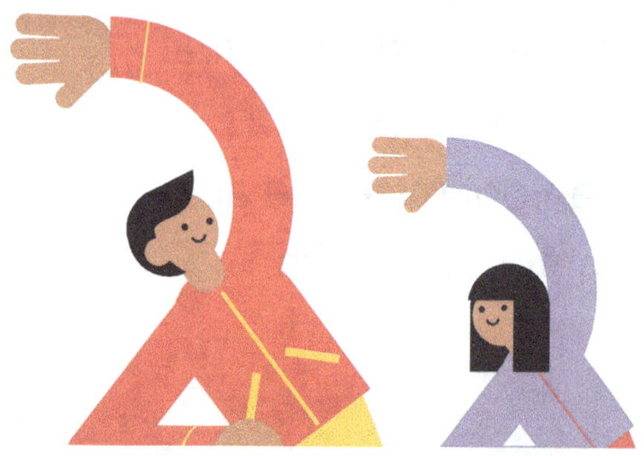

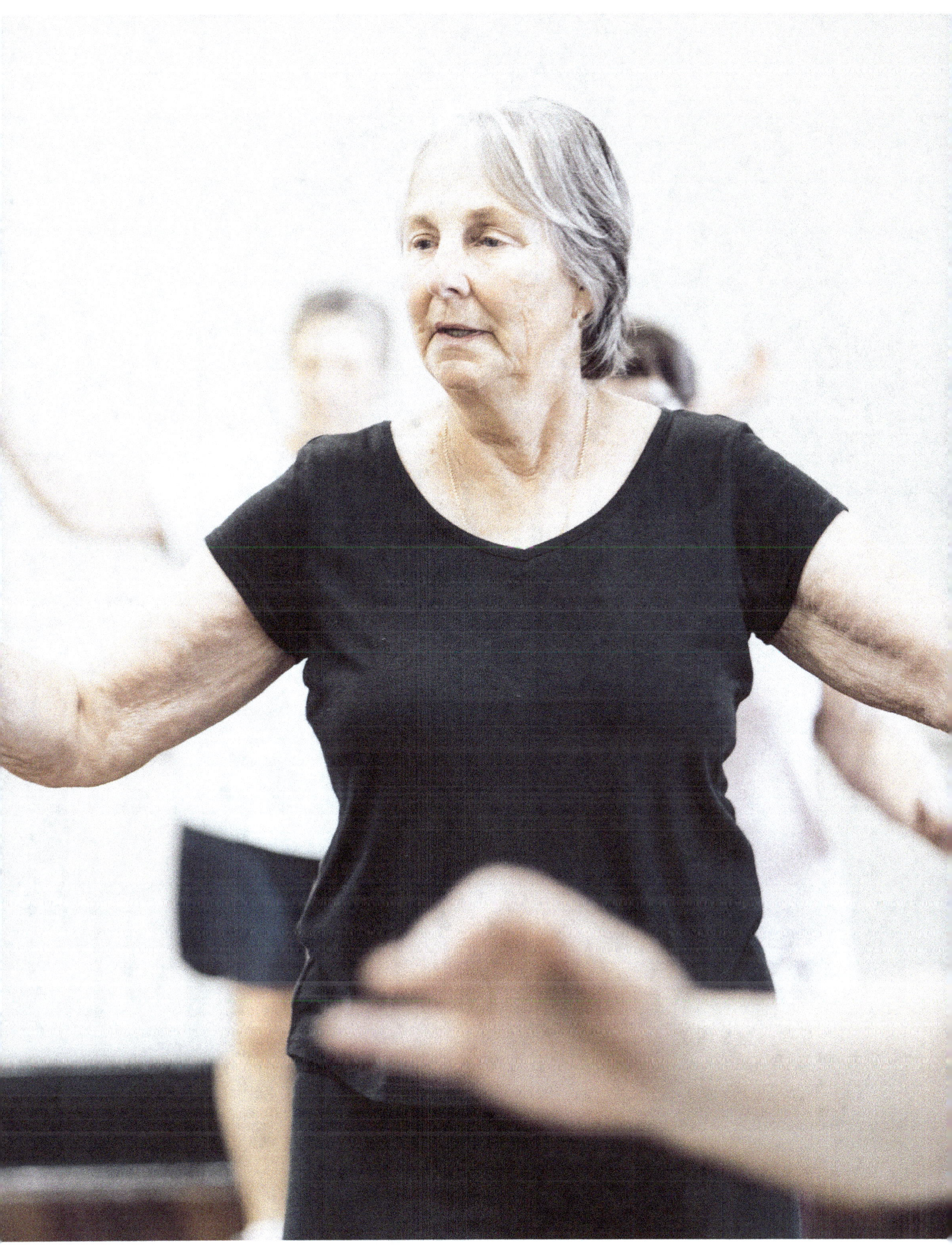

STRESS
MANAGEMENT
TECHNIQUES
FOR A CALMER,
INFLAMMATION
-FREE LIFE

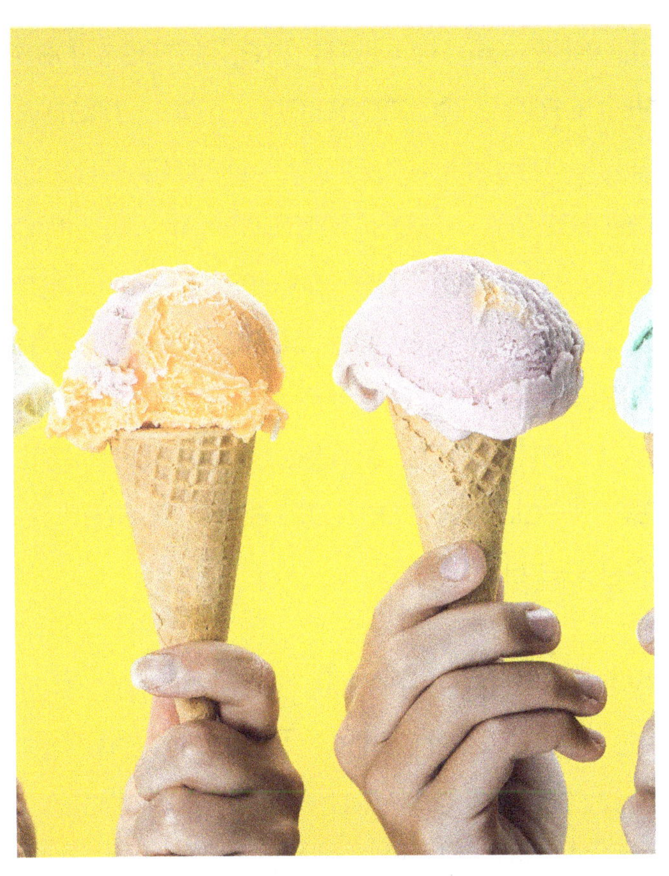

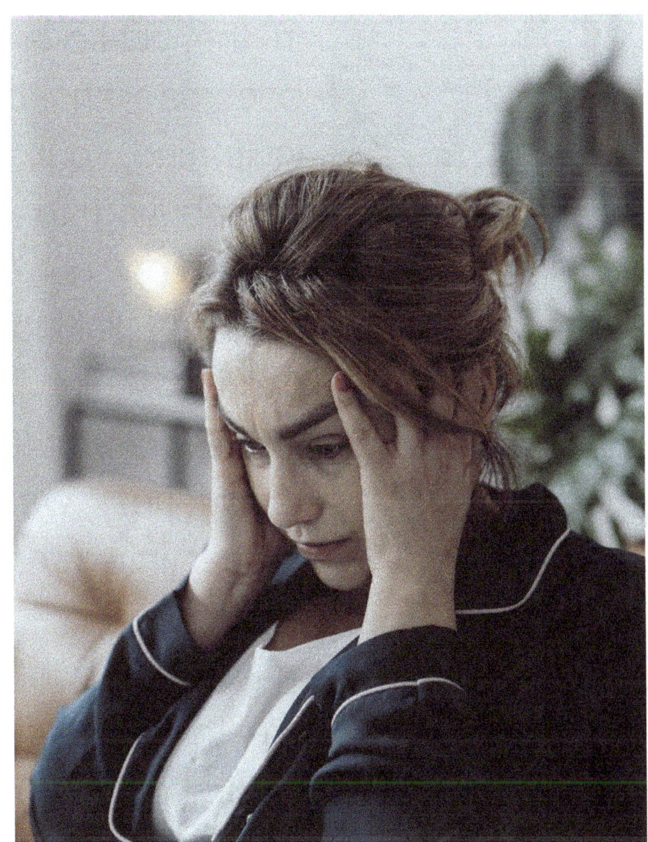

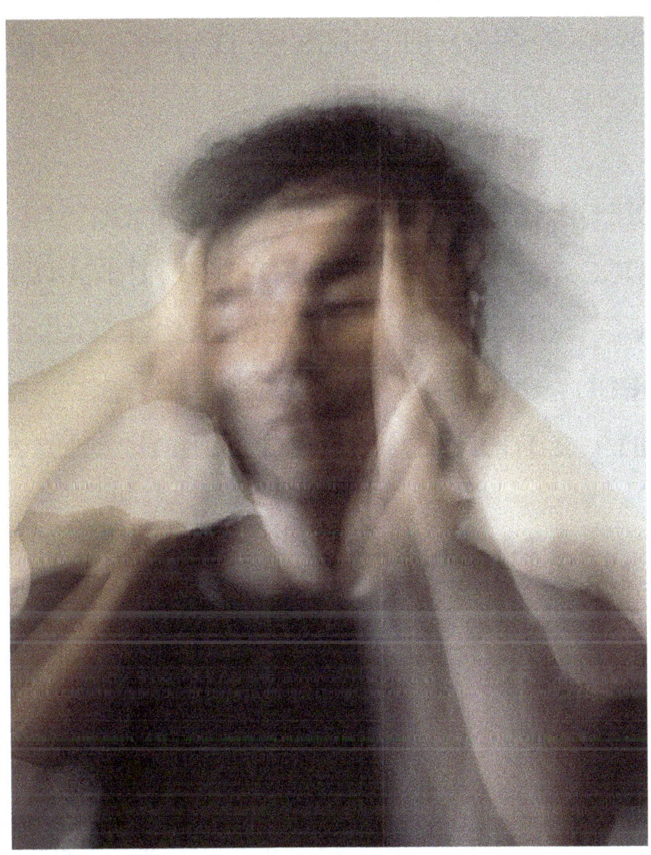

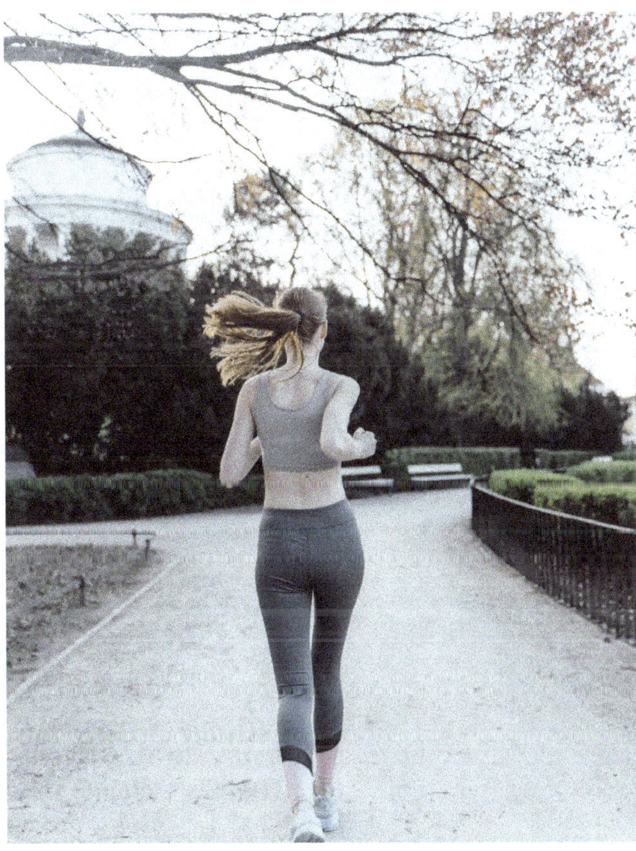

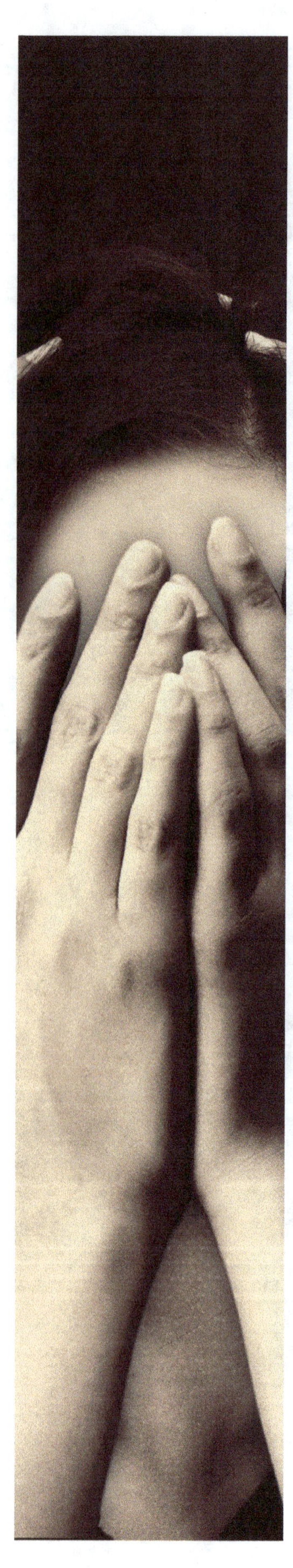

In the hustle and bustle of modern life, stress has become an unwelcome companion for many, infiltrating our daily routines and, unknowingly, contributing to inflammation. The impact of chronic stress on our health cannot be overstated, with research linking it to a range of conditions from cardiovascular issues to autoimmune disorders. However, armed with effective stress management techniques, we can reclaim control and foster a calmer, inflammation-free life.

In the chaos of daily life, the simple act of mindful breathing can serve as an anchor. Take moments throughout the day to focus on your breath, inhaling deeply and exhaling slowly. This mindful pause not only reduces stress but also initiates a physiological response that counters inflammation.

Meditation is a potent tool for stress management, offering a quiet refuge for the mind. Whether through guided sessions or self-directed practice, regular meditation has been shown to decrease stress hormones, promoting a more balanced inflammatory response.

Physical activity is a natural stress reliever that goes beyond its physical benefits. Engaging in regular exercise releases endorphins, the body's natural mood lifters, while also reducing inflammation. Find an activity you enjoy, be it yoga, jogging, or dancing, and make it a consistent part of your routine.

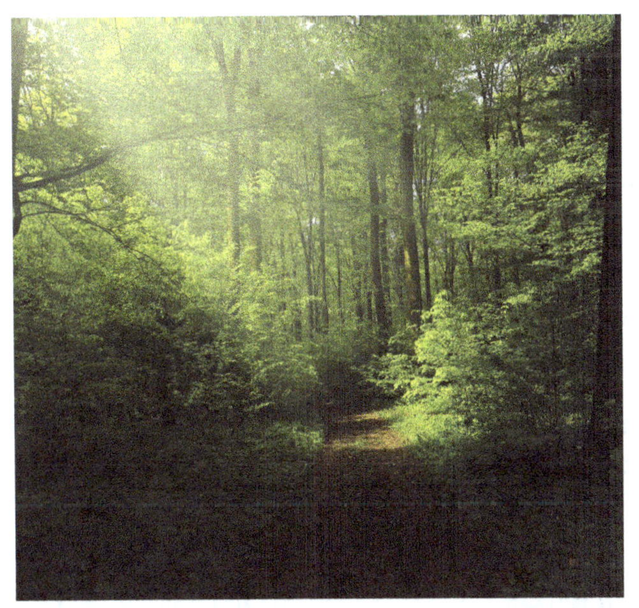

CONNECT WITH NATURE: GROUNDING FOR THE SOUL

Nature has a profound calming effect on the mind. Take moments to connect with the natural world —whether it's a walk in the park, a hike in the mountains, or simply sitting in a garden. Nature's soothing embrace has the power to alleviate stress and, consequently, reduce inflammation.

CULTIVATE A SUPPORTIVE SOCIAL NETWORK

Human connections are a powerful antidote to stress. Cultivate a supportive social network, sharing your thoughts and feelings with trusted friends or family. The emotional support derived from healthy relationships contributes to a resilient mental state, mitigating the effects of stress-induced inflammation.

PRIORITIZE SLEEP FOR RESTORATION

Adequate sleep is crucial for managing stress. To achieve this, establish a bedtime routine, create a restful sleep environment, and prioritize sufficient sleep each night. Sleep not only rejuvenates the body but also plays a pivotal role in regulating inflammation.

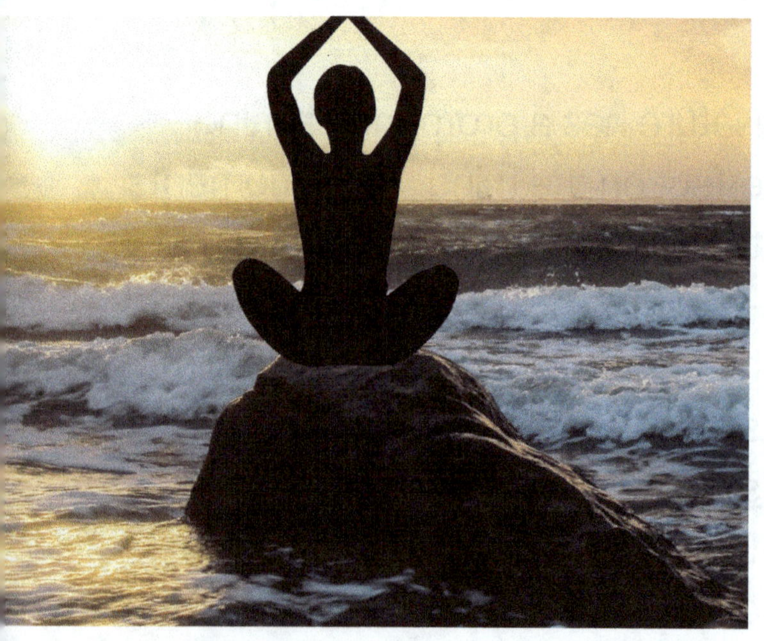

Establishing realistic goals and setting boundaries is crucial for managing stress. Learn to say no when necessary, prioritize tasks, and break them into manageable steps. This proactive approach fosters a sense of control, reducing stress and its inflammatory impact.

Mind-body practices like yoga and tai chi combine physical movement with mindfulness, offering a holistic approach to stress management. These practices not only enhance flexibility and strength but also cultivate a centered and calm mind, promoting an inflammation-free life.

Laughter truly is a potent elixir for stress. Engage in activities that bring joy and humor into your life. Whether it's watching a funny movie, attending a comedy show, or spending time with playful pets, laughter releases endorphins, promoting a positive mood and mitigating the effects of stress-induced inflammation.

Engaging in creative activities can be a therapeutic outlet for stress. Whether it's painting, writing, or playing music, creative expression provides a means to channel emotions positively, reducing the physiological toll of chronic stress on the body.

By adopting mindful practices, embracing supportive relationships, and prioritizing self-care, individuals can navigate life's challenges with grace and resilience. This can lead to a calmer, inflammation-free existence marked by well-being, vitality, and a greater sense of equilibrium.

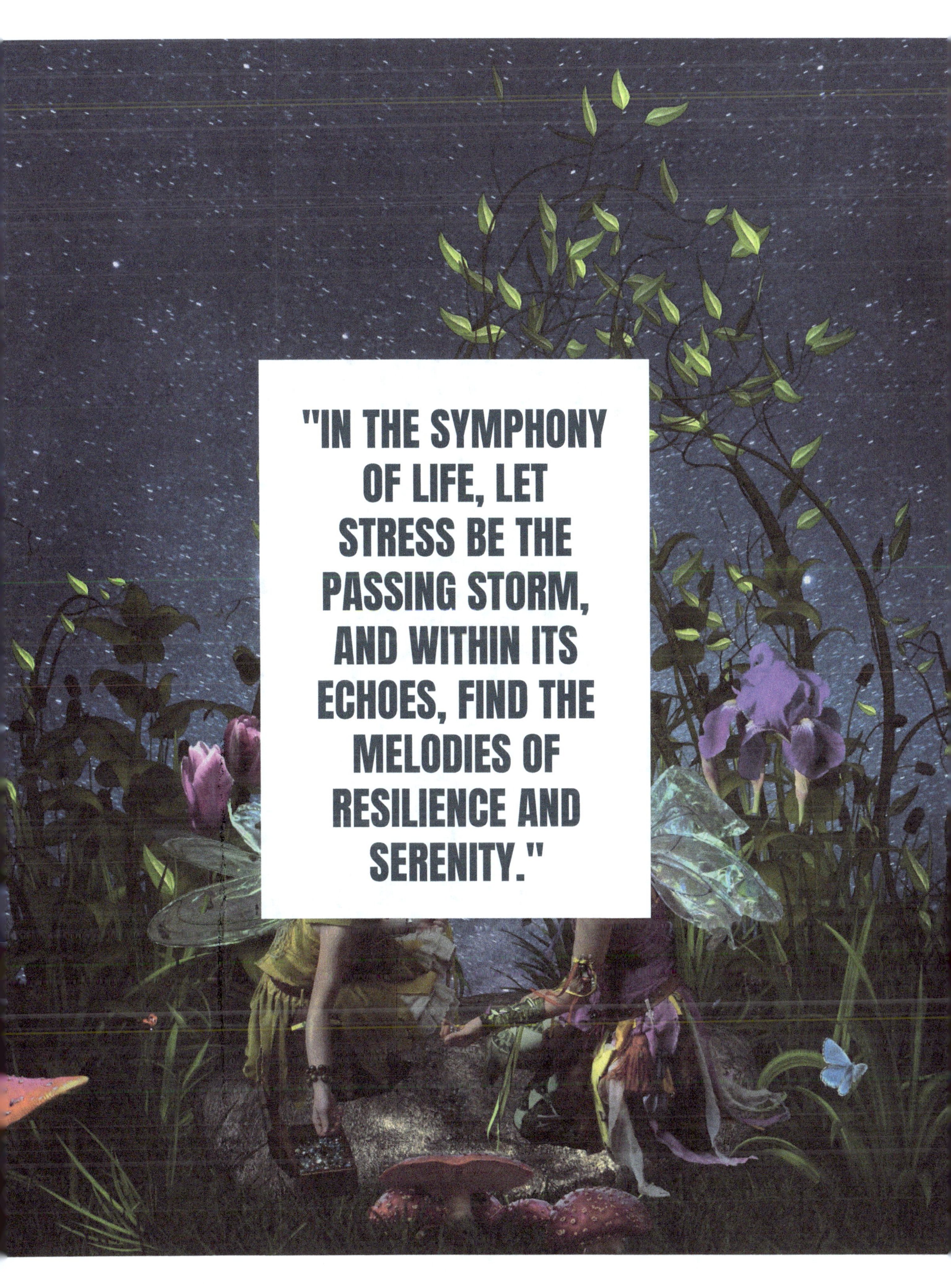
"IN THE SYMPHONY OF LIFE, LET STRESS BE THE PASSING STORM, AND WITHIN ITS ECHOES, FIND THE MELODIES OF RESILIENCE AND SERENITY."

A GUIDE TO ANTI-INFLAMMATORY SUPERFOODS

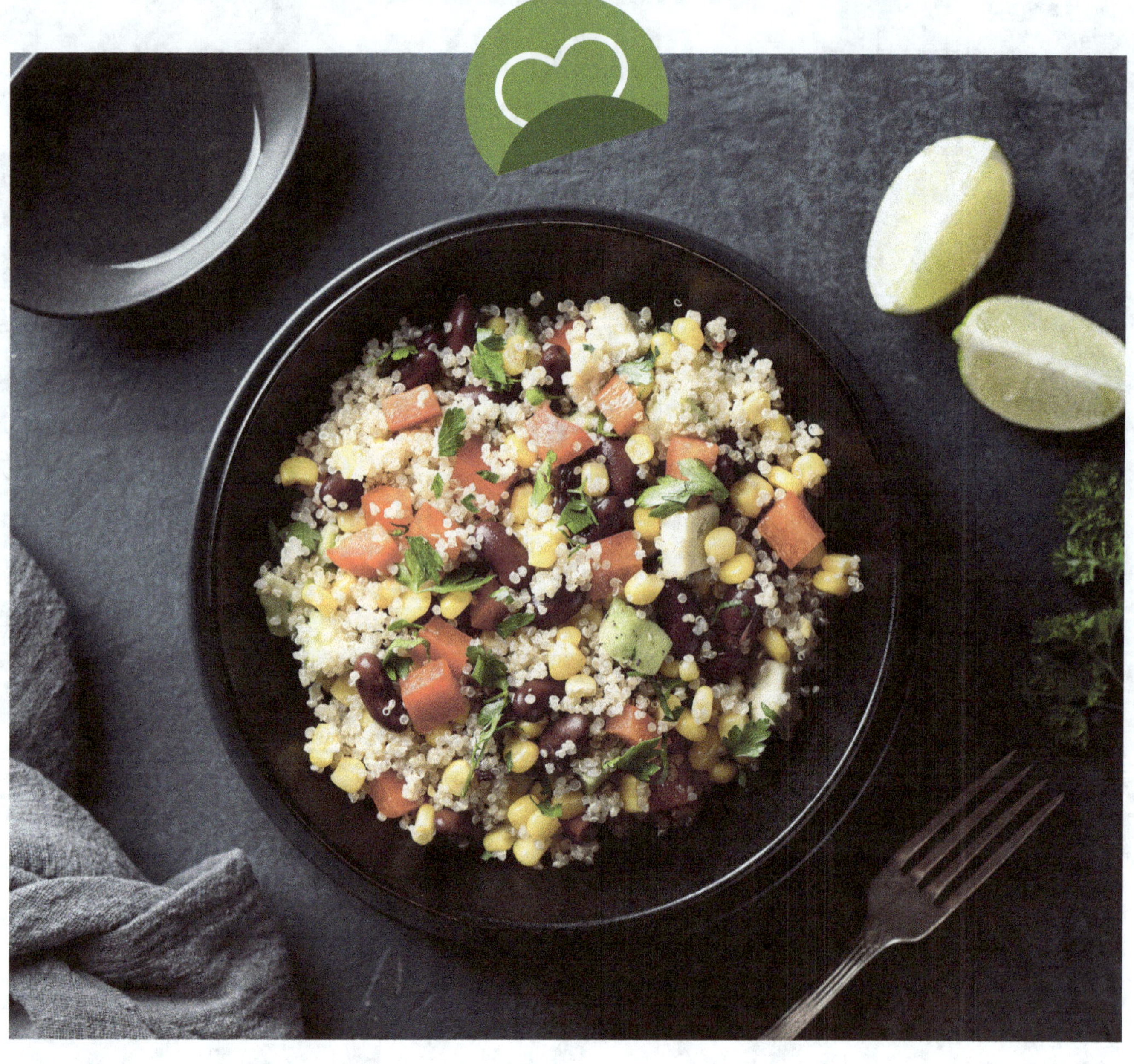

Nature offers a variety of superfoods that can help combat inflammation, a key factor in the development of chronic diseases. These foods not only taste great but also promote overall well-being. Join us on a journey through the world of anti-inflammatory superfoods.

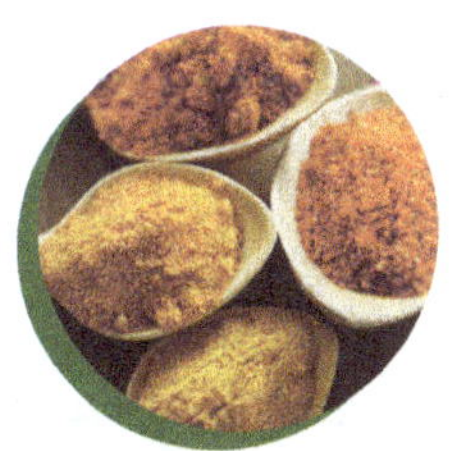

Turmeric: The Golden Healer

Turmeric is a potent anti-inflammatory spice due to its active compound curcumin. It has been widely used in traditional medicine and has demonstrated remarkable abilities to reduce inflammation and contribute to overall health. You can incorporate turmeric into your diet in curries, teas, or smoothies to take a flavorful step towards wellness.

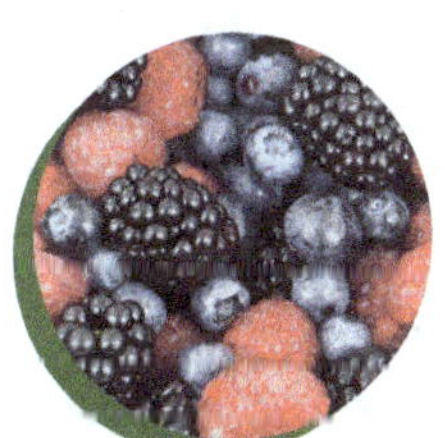

Berries: Nature's Antioxidant Gems

Berries are flavorful and rich in antioxidants, which combat oxidative stress and inflammation in the body. They can be enjoyed as a snack, added to yogurt, or blended into a refreshing smoothie. Incorporating berries into an anti-inflammatory diet is a delightful choice.

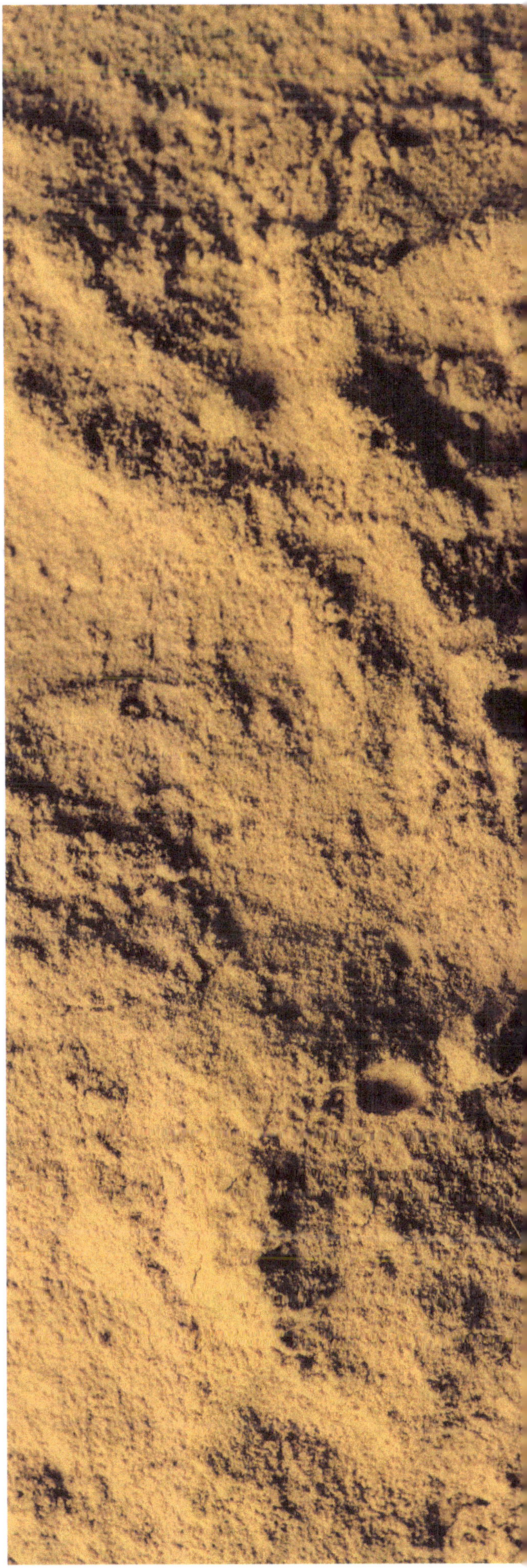

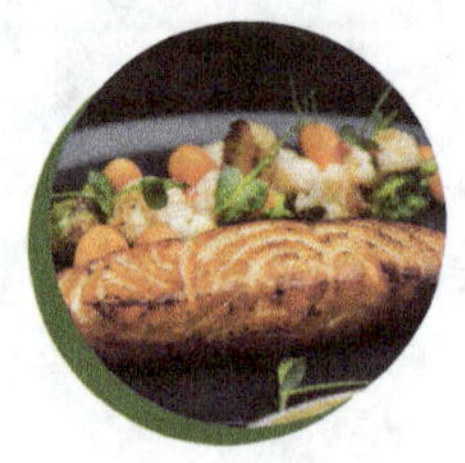

Fatty Fish: Omega-3 Powerhouses

Fatty fish like salmon, mackerel, and sardines are not only delicious but also rich in omega-3 fatty acids. These essential fats play a crucial role in reducing inflammation and supporting heart health. To harness the anti-inflammatory benefits of omega-3s, aim to include fatty fish in your diet regularly.

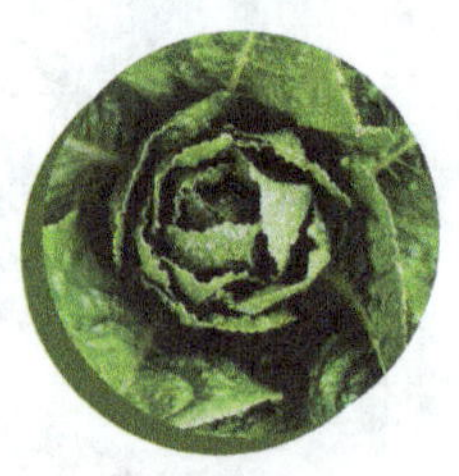

Leafy Greens: Nutrient-Rich Elegance

Incorporating dark, leafy greens like kale, spinach, and Swiss chard into your diet is a wise choice. These greens are packed with vitamins, minerals, and antioxidants that contribute to overall health. Additionally, their anti-inflammatory properties make them a staple in promoting well-being. You can enjoy them in salads, smoothies, or sautés.

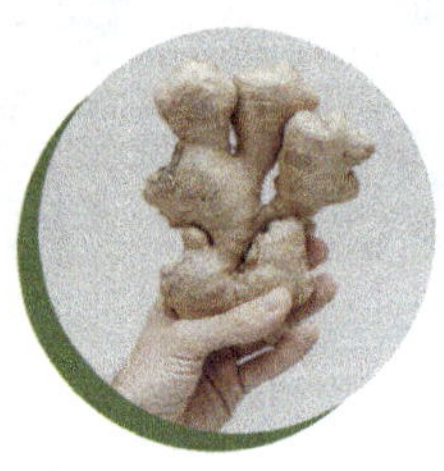

Ginger: A Zest for Life

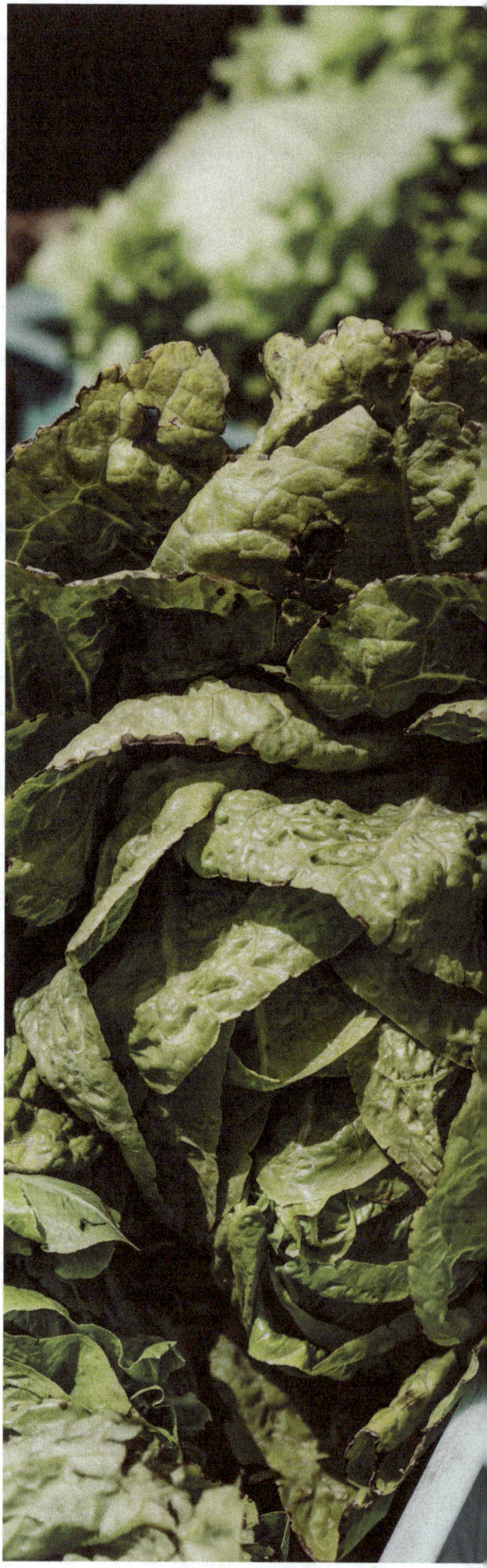

Ginger is a versatile root with potent anti-inflammatory and antioxidant properties. Its zesty flavor is well-known. It adds a burst of flavor to tea, stir-fries, and various dishes while contributing to your body's defense against inflammation.

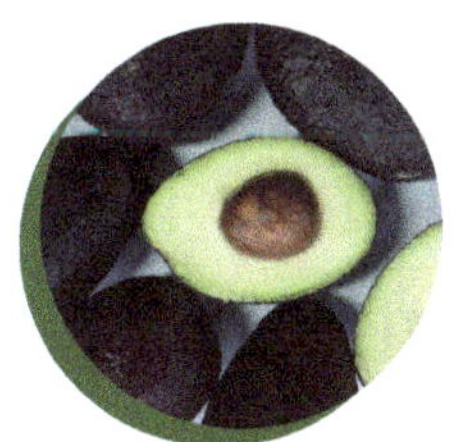

Avocado: Creamy Goodness with Benefits

Avocados are creamy, nutrient-rich, and delicious. They are also effective in fighting inflammation due to their high content of monounsaturated fats and antioxidants. You can enjoy avocados on toast, in salads, or as the star ingredient in guacamole.

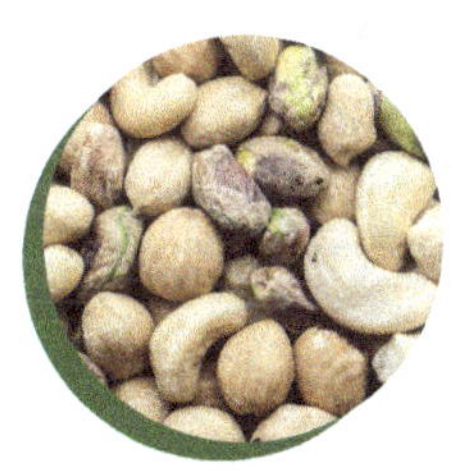

Nuts and Seeds: Bite-Sized Nutrition

Almonds, walnuts, chia seeds, and flaxseeds are nutritional powerhouses. They are rich in omega-3 fatty acids, fiber, and antioxidants, which help reduce inflammation. You can sprinkle them on yogurt, blend them into smoothies, or enjoy them as a wholesome snack.

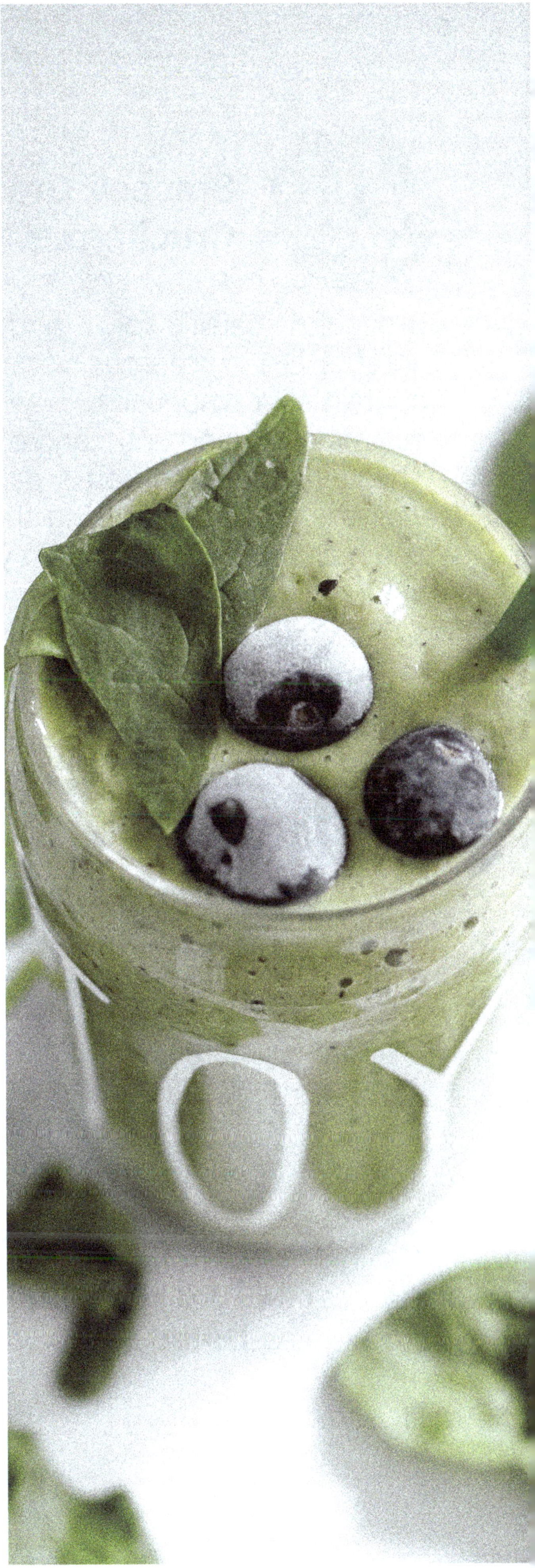

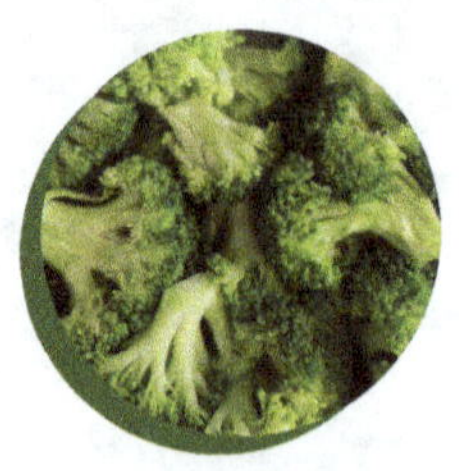

Broccoli: Green Cruciferous Warrior

Broccoli, cauliflower, and Brussels sprouts are cruciferous vegetables that contain compounds with anti-inflammatory and anti-cancer properties. These vegetables are packed with vitamins and fiber, making them a tasty and nutritious way to support your body's natural defense against inflammation.

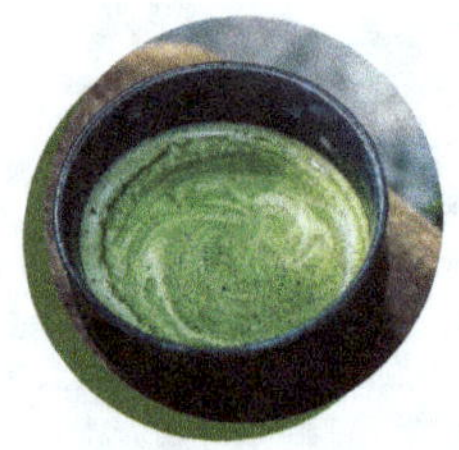

Green Tea: Sip Your Way to Wellness

Green tea is a beverage that contains antioxidants, including catechins, which are known for their anti-inflammatory properties. To stay hydrated and benefit from its inflammation-fighting properties, replace sugary drinks with a cup of green tea.

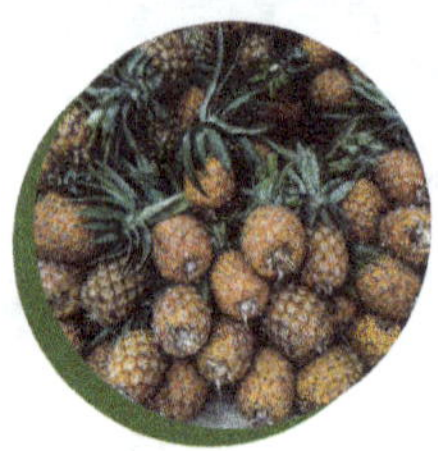

Pineapple: Tropical Anti-Inflammatory Delight

Pineapple contains bromelain, an enzyme with anti-inflammatory properties. It adds a sweet and tangy twist to your diet while providing a natural means to combat inflammation. You can enjoy pineapple on its own, in fruit salads, or as a refreshing addition to smoothies.

Incorporating these anti-inflammatory superfoods into your daily meals not only enhances the flavor of your diet but also empowers you on your journey toward optimal health. Nature has given us a colorful variety of foods that not only satisfy our taste buds but also support our pursuit of a healthy and energetic life.

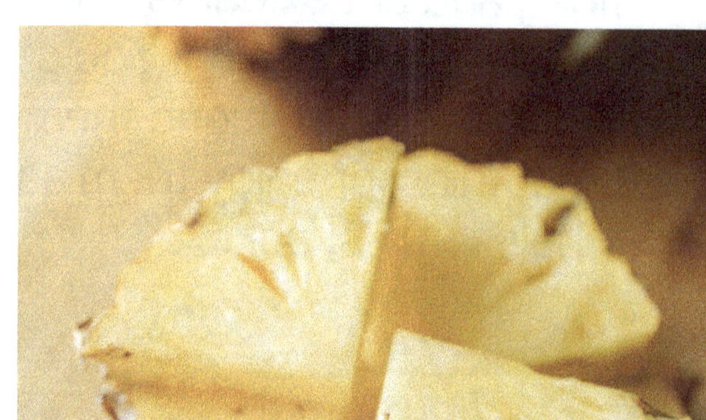

THE LINK BETWEEN INFLAMMATION AND REST

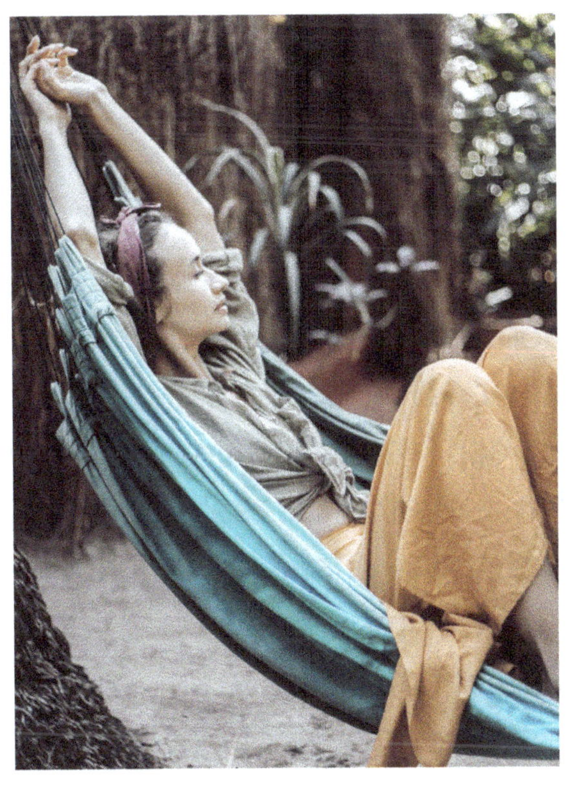

The Sleep-Inflammation Interplay: A Nightly Balancing Act

Quality sleep is essential for the body's repair and restoration process. During deep sleep, the immune system releases cytokines, which help combat inflammation. Insufficient or disrupted sleep can disrupt this delicate balance, leading to an overactive inflammatory response. Therefore, it is crucial to prioritize rest as a cornerstone of inflammation management.

In contemporary life, rest is often overlooked due to work, family, and other responsibilities. However, recent research shows a strong connection between inflammation and rest, emphasizing the importance of quality rest for our overall health.

Understanding Inflammation's Toll on the Body

Inflammation is the body's natural response to injury, infection, or stress. Acute inflammation is necessary and protective, but chronic inflammation can be destructive. It has been linked to various health issues, from cardiovascular diseases to autoimmune conditions. Lifestyle factors influence the body's ability to regulate inflammation, and quality rest is crucial in this process.

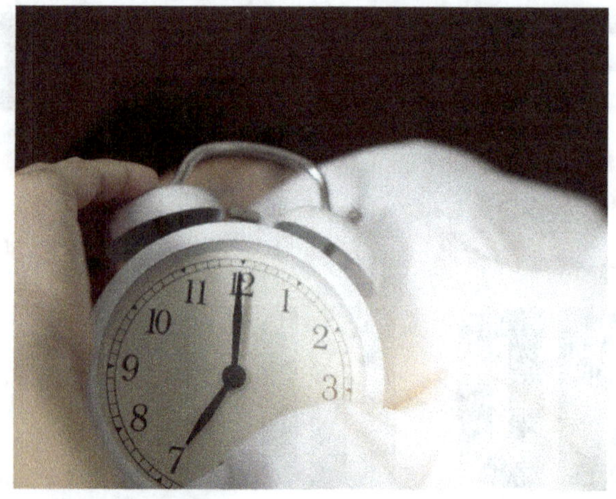

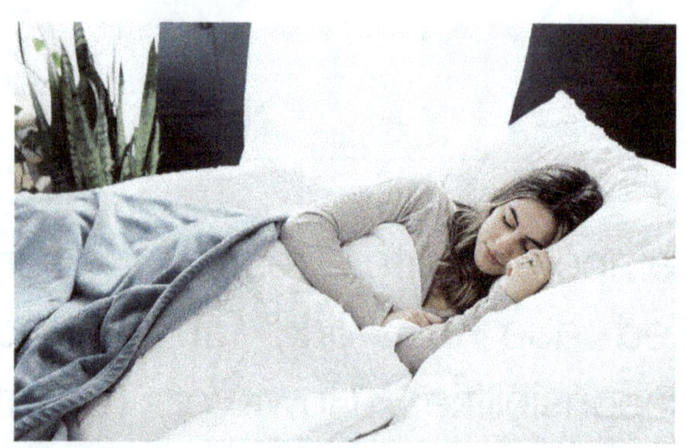

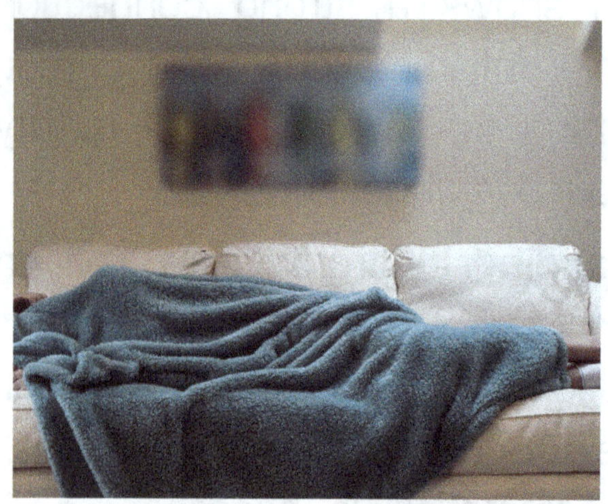

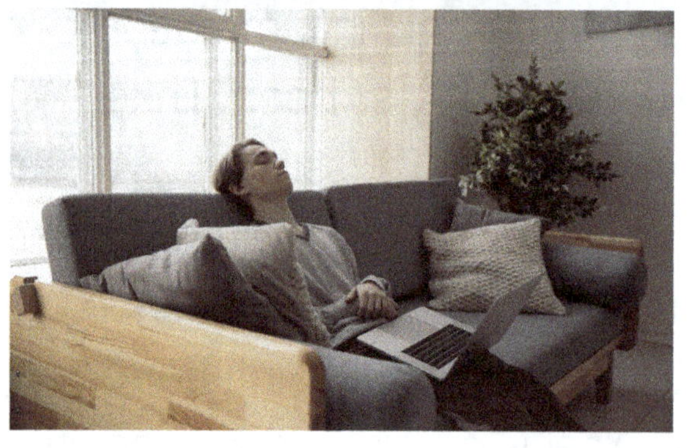

Cortisol, Stress, and the Sleep Cycle: A Tangled Web

Cortisol, a stress hormone, is linked to the body's response to stress and also affects sleep and inflammation. Disruptions in the circadian rhythm, often caused by irregular sleep patterns, can lead to abnormal cortisol secretion. Elevated cortisol levels can contribute to increased inflammation. Therefore, it is important to maintain consistent and restorative sleep to balance these physiological processes.

Practical Strategies for Enhancing Rest and Managing Inflammation

Recognizing the interdependence of rest and inflammation opens avenues for proactive health management. To contribute to improved sleep quality, establish a consistent sleep schedule, create a conducive sleep environment, and practice relaxation techniques before bedtime. Additionally, adopting stress management practices, such as meditation and deep breathing exercises, can support both quality rest and inflammation reduction.

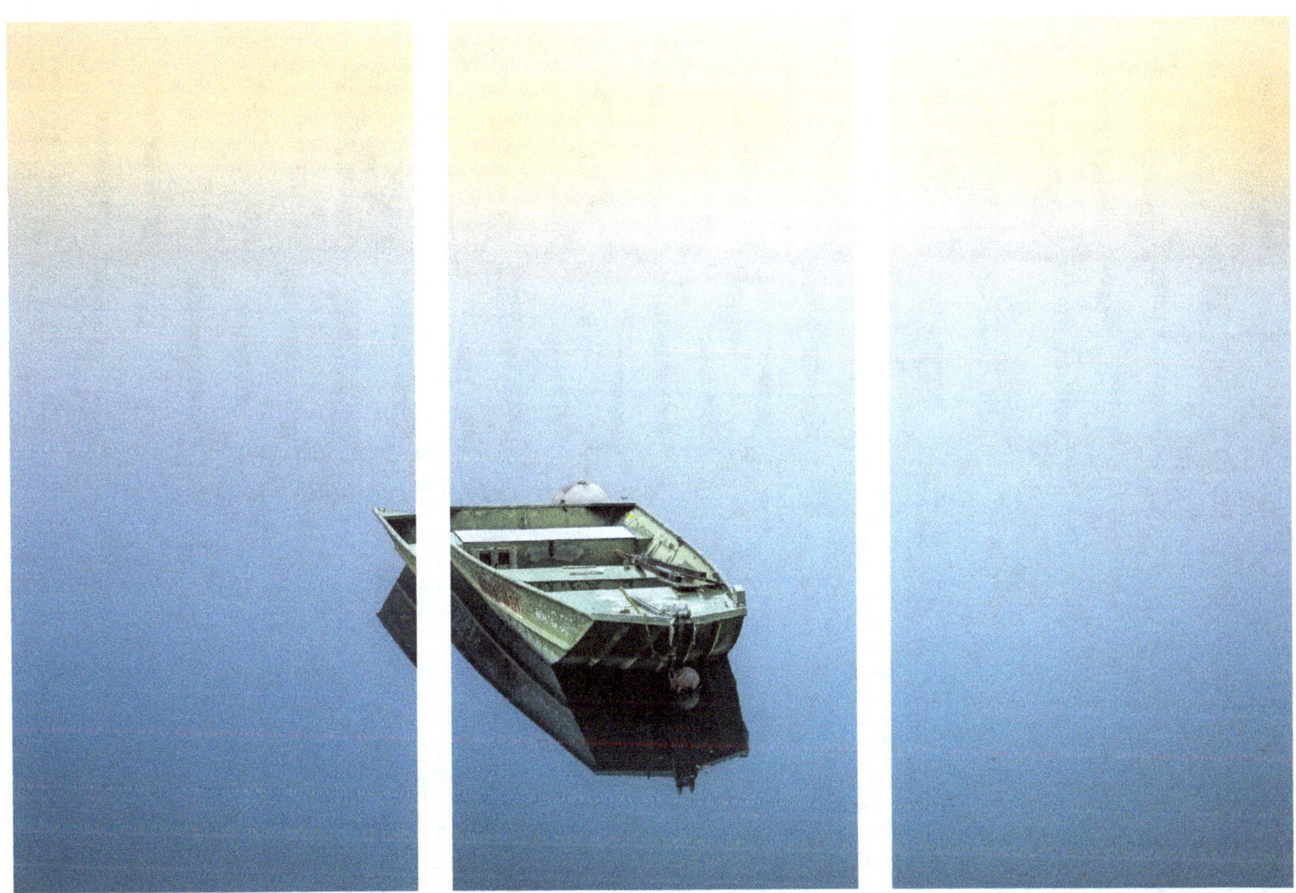

The Mind-Body Connection: Mental Well-Being and Inflammation

The link between mental well-being and inflammation is increasingly acknowledged beyond the physical realm. Chronic stress, anxiety, and depression can contribute to an inflammatory milieu in the body if left unaddressed. Therefore, rest becomes a vital component of self-care and a potent ally in nurturing mental well-being, fostering a positive impact on overall inflammation levels.

Nurturing Health through Restful Reverie

Inflammation and rest are closely connected in maintaining good health. It is essential to prioritize and honor the need for sufficient, quality rest. Rest is not a luxury but a fundamental pillar of well-being. In modern life, it is wise to allow our bodies the restful reverie they crave. This sanctuary keeps inflammation in check and rekindles vitality with each night's rest.

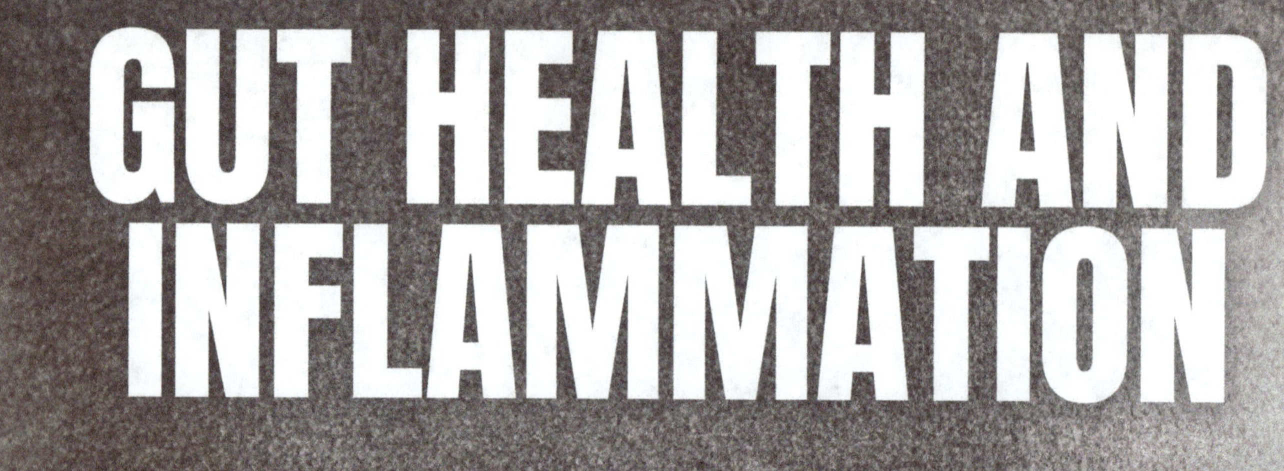

GUT HEALTH AND INFLAMMATION

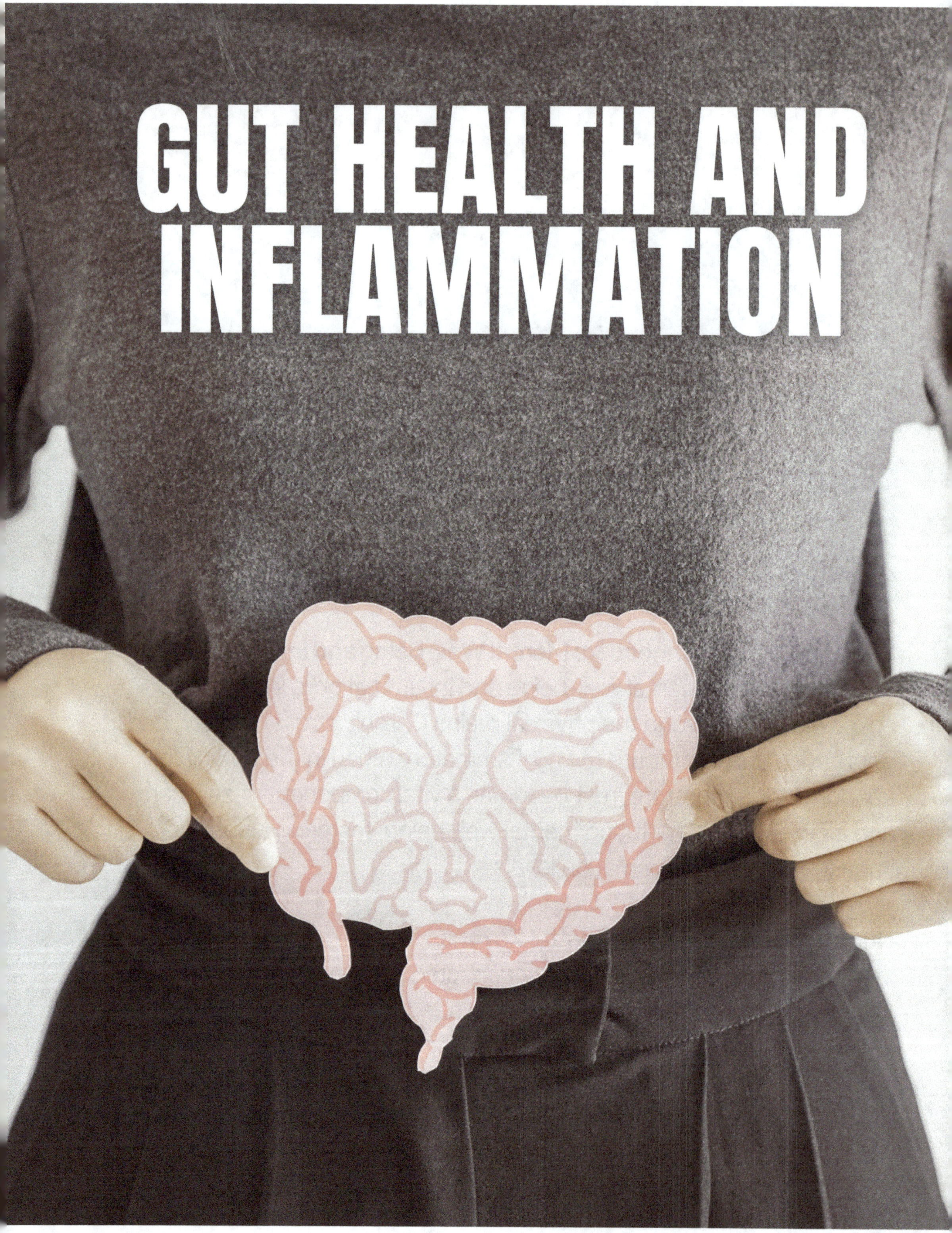

BODY'S RESPONSE

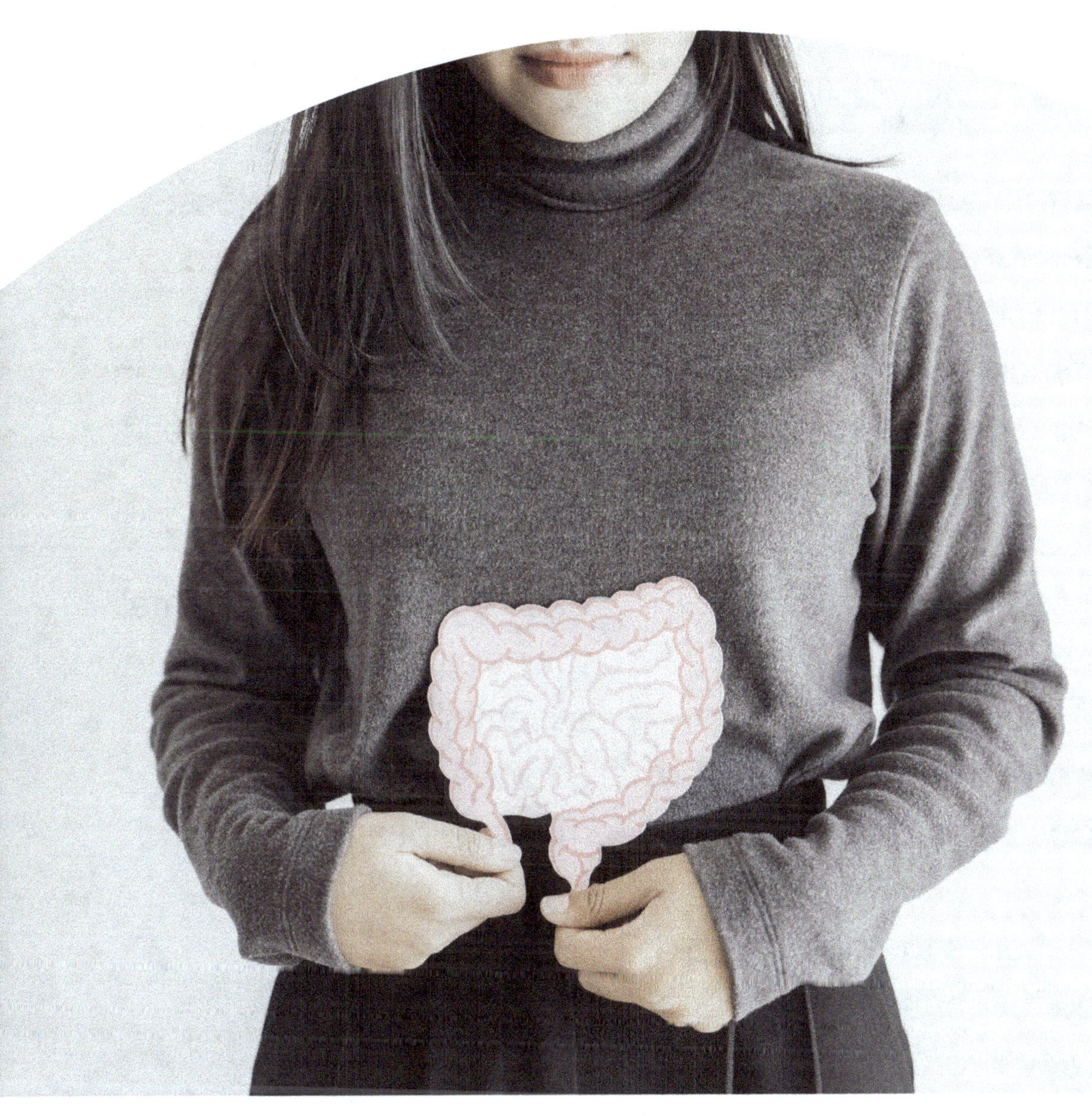

The Inflammatory Players: Cells and Chemicals at Work

Inflammation involves cells and chemicals working together to combat a threat. The immune system's white blood cells rush to the affected area to neutralize invaders. Chemicals such as cytokines and prostaglandins help coordinate this response by signaling cells and regulating the process.

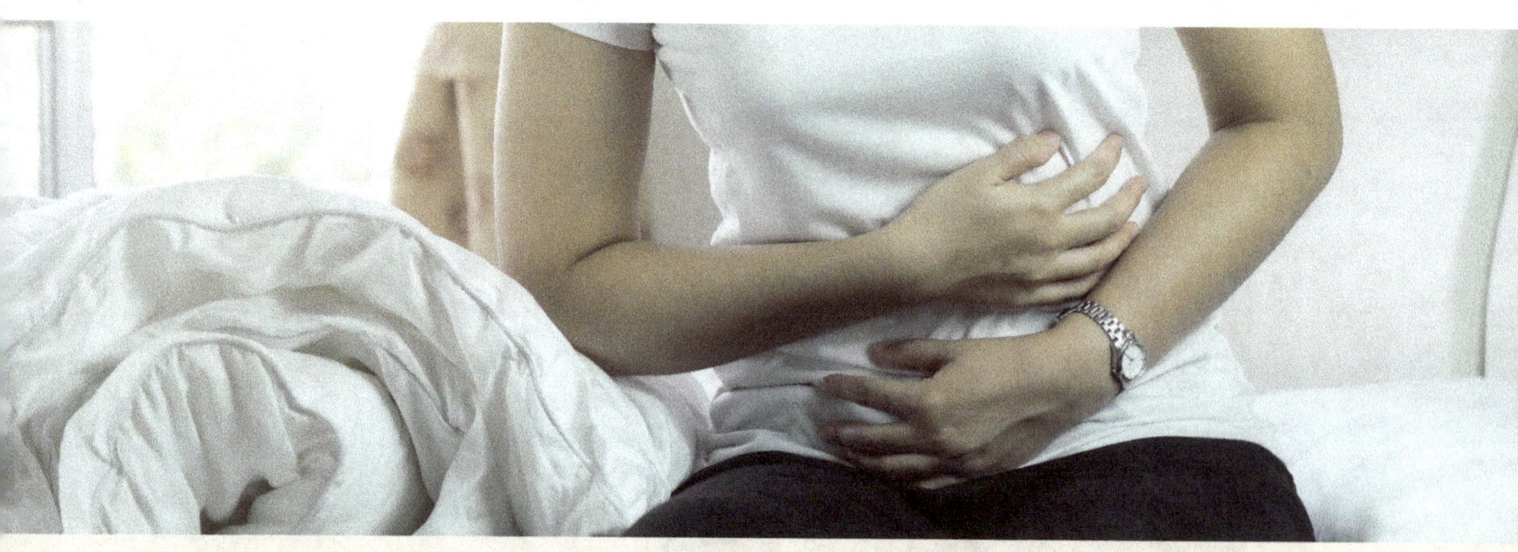

Signs of Inflammation: Red Flags and Protective Measures

Recognizing the signs of inflammation is crucial. Common signs include redness, swelling, heat, and pain. These are protective measures that isolate the affected area, eliminate the cause of cell injury, and initiate the repair process.

Acute vs. Chronic Inflammation: The Timely Response and Lingering Threats

Acute inflammation is the body's rapid and short-lived response to injury or infection. It is a well-orchestrated process aimed at resolving the issue. In contrast, chronic inflammation is persistent and can become harmful, contributing to conditions such as arthritis, heart disease, and diabetes.

Inflammatory Triggers: Culprits in the Modern Lifestyle

Certain lifestyle factors can trigger chronic inflammation. Unhealthy diets, lack of exercise, stress, and exposure to environmental toxins all play a role. It is essential to make informed choices in these areas to manage inflammation and maintain overall health.

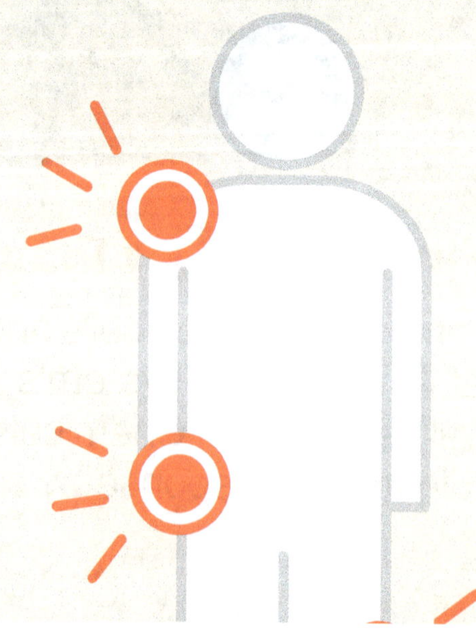

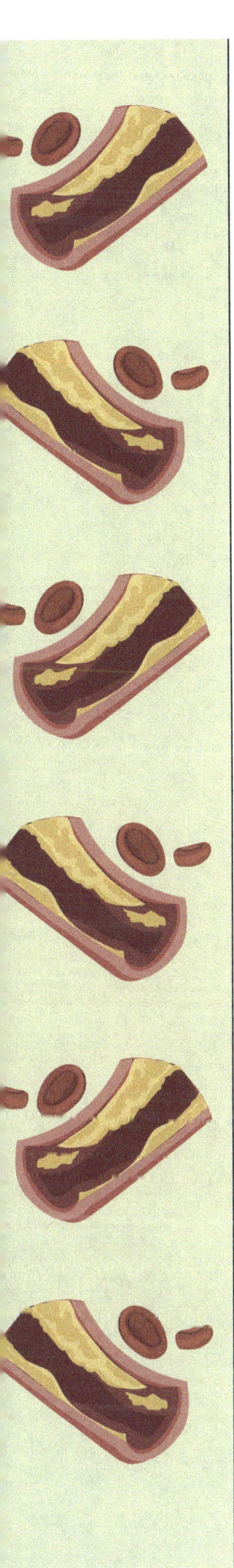

Gut Health and Inflammation: The Digestive Connection

The gut plays a crucial role in inflammation. Imbalanced gut bacteria can contribute to chronic inflammation. A diet rich in fiber, probiotics, and prebiotics can help nurture a healthy gut environment, positively influencing the inflammatory response.

Anti-Inflammatory Lifestyle: Your Defense Strategy

To adopt an anti-inflammatory lifestyle, make choices that reduce inflammation. This includes maintaining a balanced diet that is rich in fruits, vegetables, and omega-3 fatty acids, engaging in regular exercise, managing stress, getting enough sleep, and avoiding tobacco and excessive alcohol. These lifestyle adjustments collectively contribute to a healthier inflammatory balance.

Inflammation and Aging: A Natural Process with Management Strategies

As we get older, our body's ability to regulate inflammation may change. Age-related conditions are often associated with chronic inflammation. However, making lifestyle choices such as eating a nutrient-rich diet, exercising regularly, and managing stress can help promote healthy aging and reduce the impact of inflammation.

Inflammation and Disease: Connecting the Dots

Chronic inflammation is associated with several diseases, including heart disease, diabetes, cancer, and neurodegenerative conditions, which may have inflammatory components. It is essential to take proactive health measures to manage inflammation and reduce the risk of developing these diseases.

Balancing Act: Harnessing the Power of Inflammation

Inflammation can be both helpful and harmful, so it's important to maintain a balance. Understanding the body's complex inflammatory response can help you make choices that promote a healthy balance. Adopting an anti-inflammatory lifestyle can lead to improved well-being, resilience, and vitality.

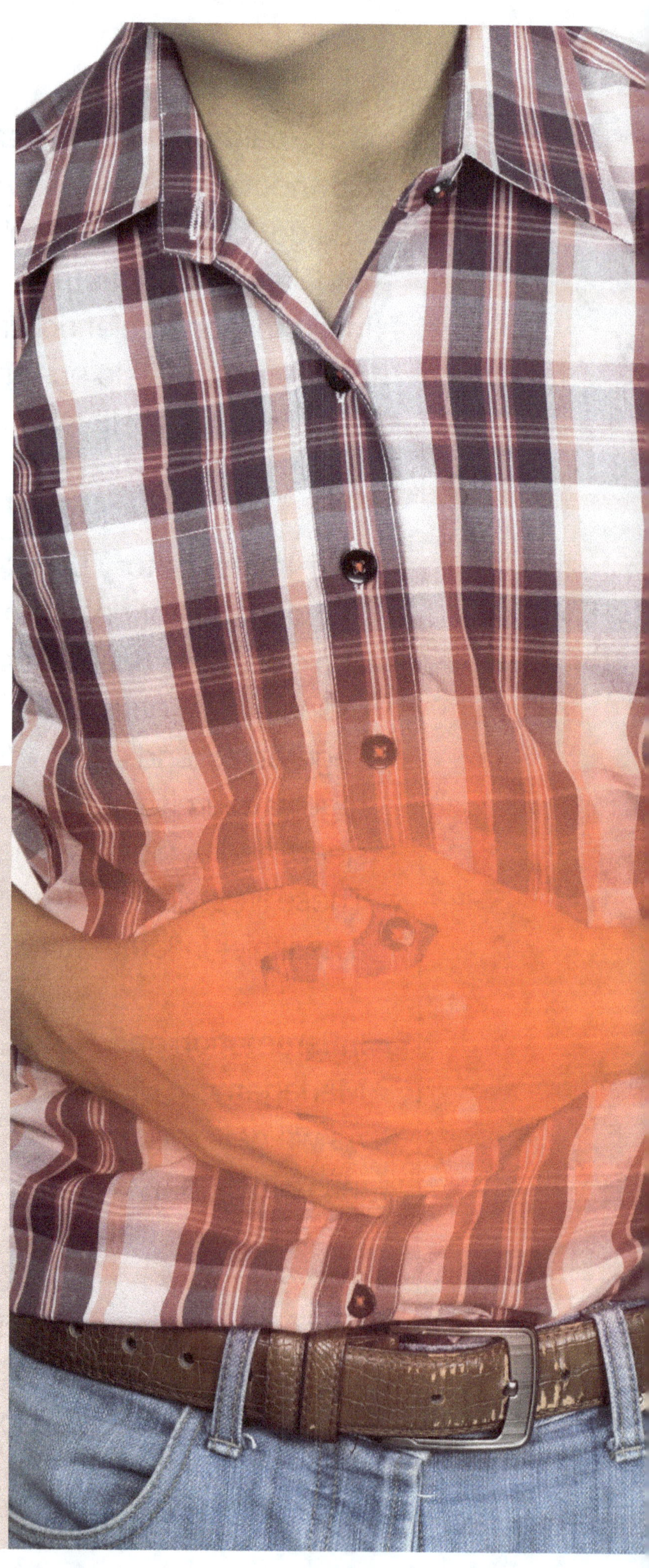

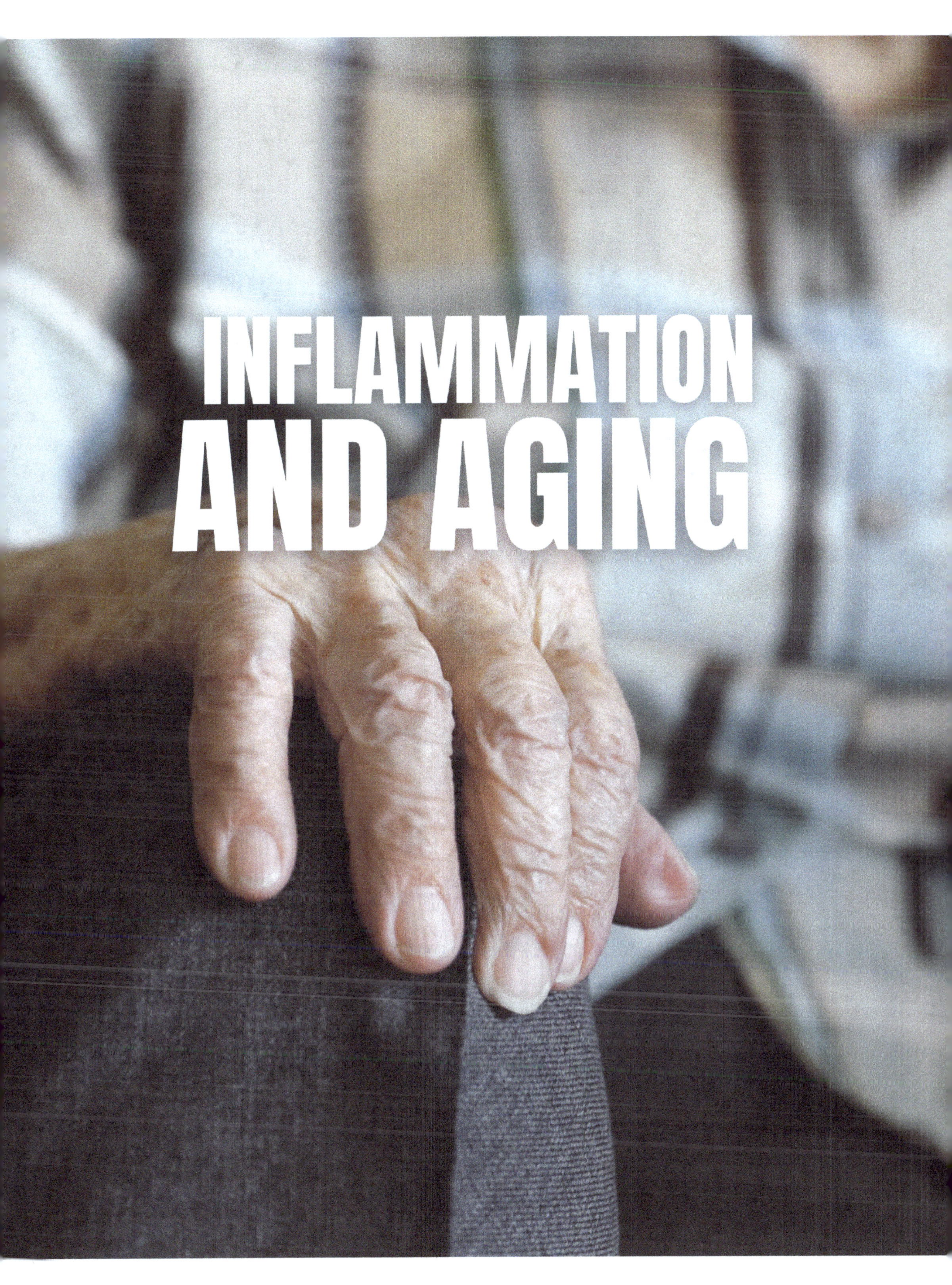
INFLAMMATION
AND AGING

AGING
INFLAMMATION
ALL OVER
AGAIN
INFLAMMATION

NAVIGATING THE AGING PROCESS: UNRAVELING THE RELATIONSHIP BETWEEN INFLAMMATION AND AGING

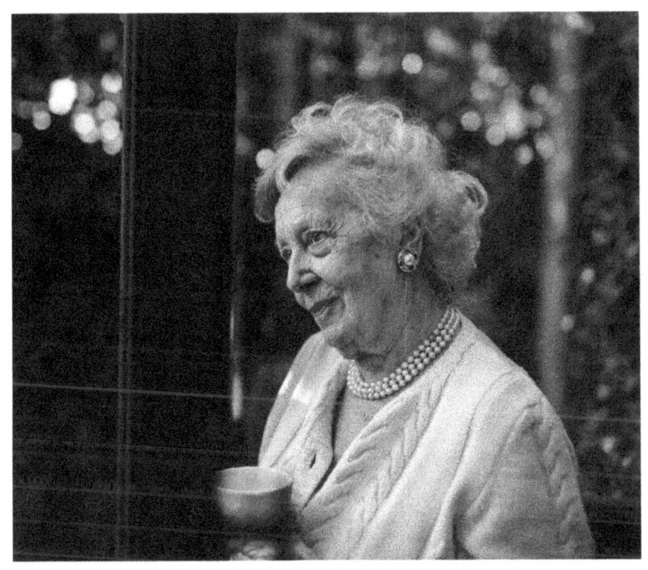

The Dynamics of Aging: A Symphony of Changes

As we age, our bodies undergo many changes. Our once-efficient repair and maintenance systems may gradually decline. Cells may not replicate as quickly, and our immune system, which defends against external threats, may show signs of wear and tear. In this intricate dance of aging, inflammation plays a role as both a protector and a potential disruptor.

Aging is a natural and inevitable aspect of life. It is marked by physical and biological changes. Inflammation is a notable player in this process. It influences the trajectory of aging and the development of age-related conditions. Let's explore the relationship between inflammation and aging. We will see how these factors shape our health as we age.

Chronic Inflammation and Aging: A Risky Partnership

Although inflammation is a crucial aspect of the body's defense mechanism, chronic inflammation presents unique challenges as we age. Chronic inflammation's subtle, persistent flame can contribute to the development and progression of various age-related conditions, from cardiovascular issues to neurodegenerative diseases. The links between chronic inflammation and the aging process are becoming increasingly evident.

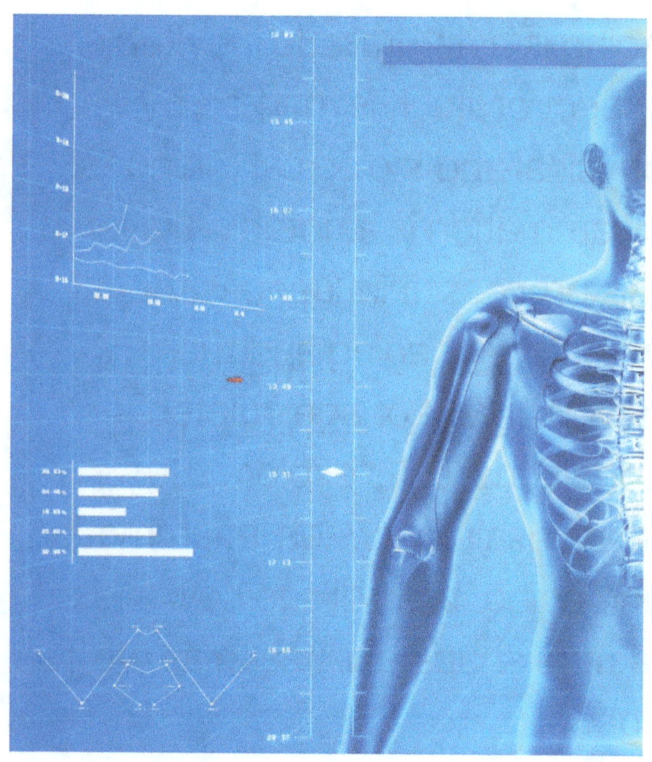

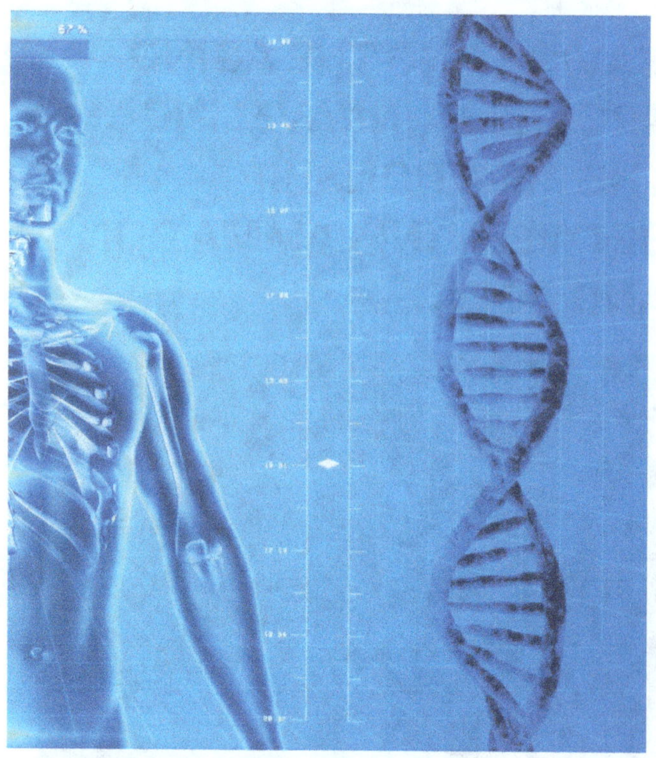

The Cellular Culprits: Senescence and Inflammaging

Cellular senescence and inflammaging are two key players in the inflammation and aging narrative. Cellular senescence refers to the state where cells cease to divide, accumulating over time and contributing to tissue dysfunction. Inflammaging, on the other hand, is a chronic, low-grade inflammation observed in aging individuals. These processes are intertwined and reinforce each other, creating an environment conducive to age-related diseases.

Inflammation's Impact on Tissues and Organs

As we age, inflammation can have a significant impact on our tissues and organs. Chronic inflammation can compromise the integrity of blood vessels, which can contribute to cardiovascular issues. Additionally, it may play a role in the deterioration of joint tissues, leading to conditions such as arthritis. It is crucial to understand these connections to develop strategies that promote healthy aging and mitigate the impact of inflammation on vital bodily systems.

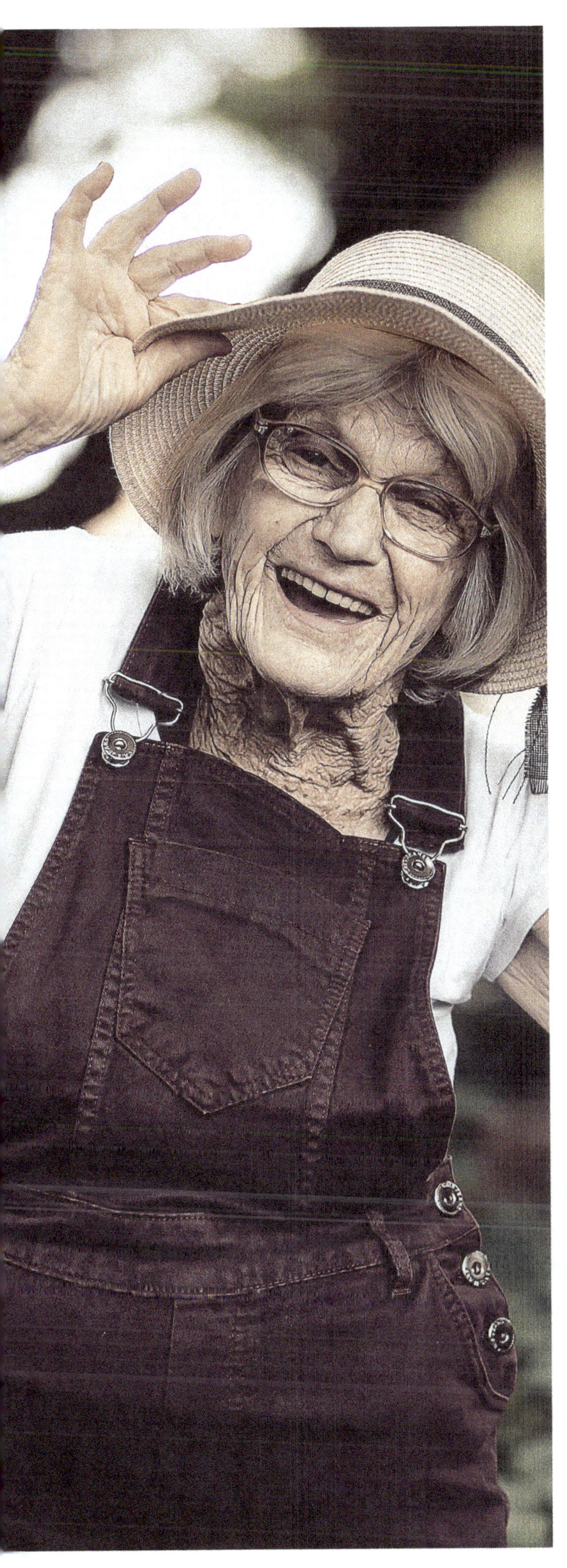

Lifestyle Choices and Inflammation: Shaping the Aging Journey

Although aging is inevitable, our lifestyle choices significantly impact how we age. Diet, exercise, stress management, and sleep all affect inflammation and can influence the aging process. To age gracefully and maintain vitality and resilience, it is essential to adopt an anti-inflammatory lifestyle.

Nutrition as a Weapon: Anti-Inflammatory Foods for Healthy Aging

In the quest for healthy aging, a nutrient-rich diet abundant in anti-inflammatory foods is essential. Incorporating fruits, vegetables, whole grains, and omega-3 fatty acids provides the necessary nutrients to counteract inflammation. This dietary strategy not only supports overall health but also becomes a powerful ally in the fight against age-related inflammation.

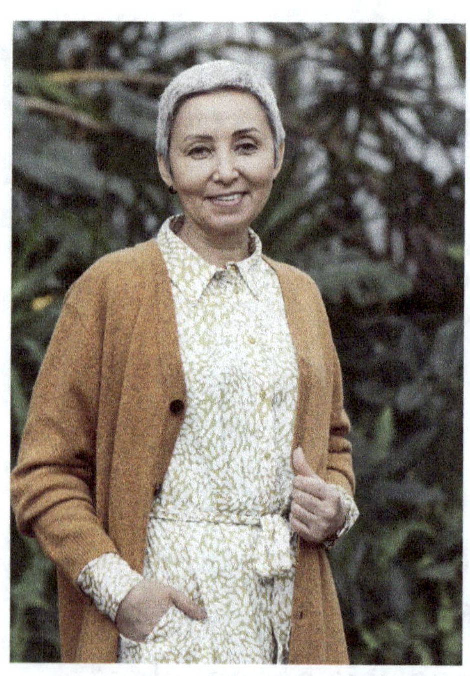

The Fountain of Youth for Body and Mind

Regular physical activity is a powerful tool for healthy aging. Exercise helps maintain physical function and has anti-inflammatory effects. There are many types of exercise, including cardiovascular, strength training, and flexibility routines, that can promote vitality and manage inflammation throughout the aging process.

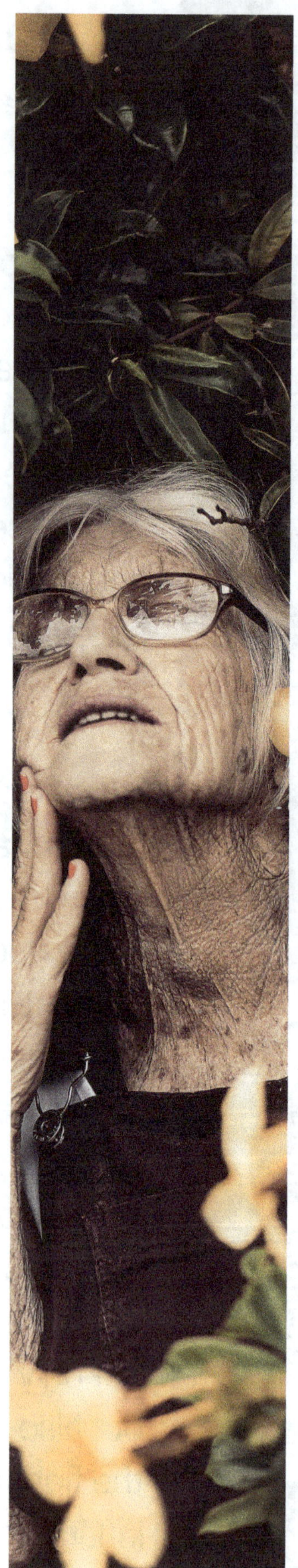

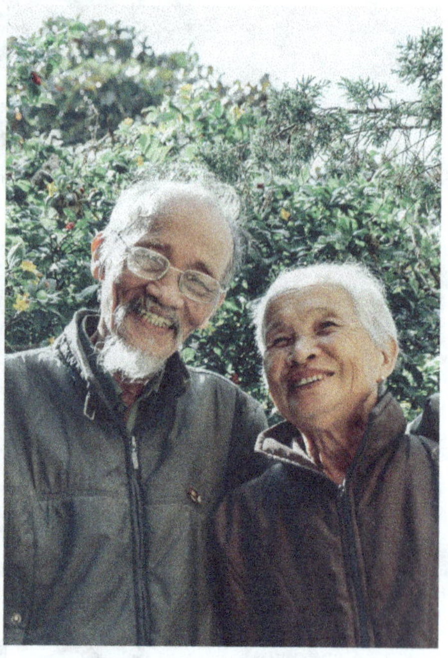

Stress Management and Emotional Well-Being

The psychological aspects of aging are closely linked to the physical. Chronic stress, anxiety, and depression can cause inflammation and speed up the aging process. To age gracefully, it is important to manage stress, maintain social connections, and prioritize emotional well-being.

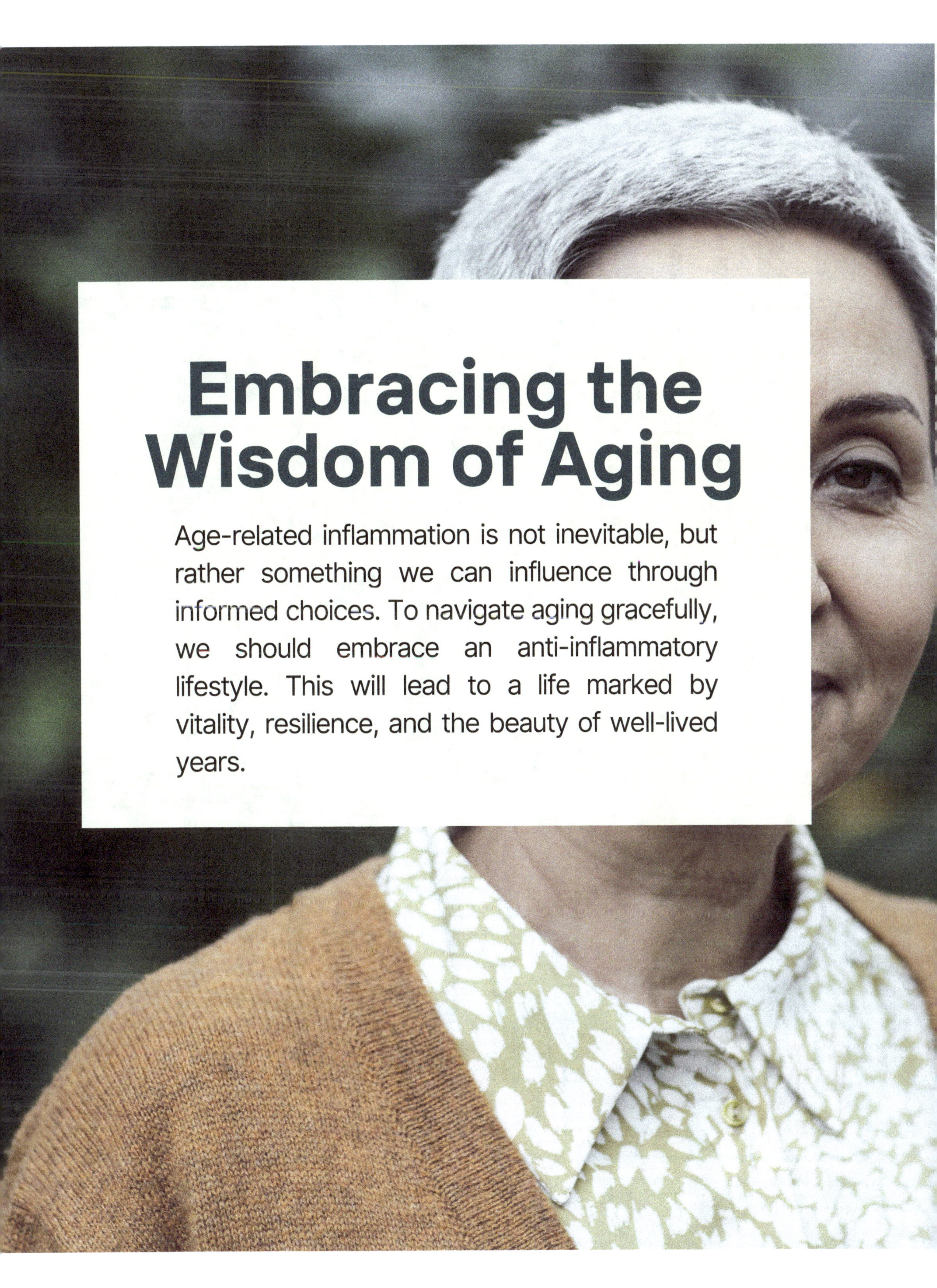

Embracing the Wisdom of Aging

Age-related inflammation is not inevitable, but rather something we can influence through informed choices. To navigate aging gracefully, we should embrace an anti-inflammatory lifestyle. This will lead to a life marked by vitality, resilience, and the beauty of well-lived years.

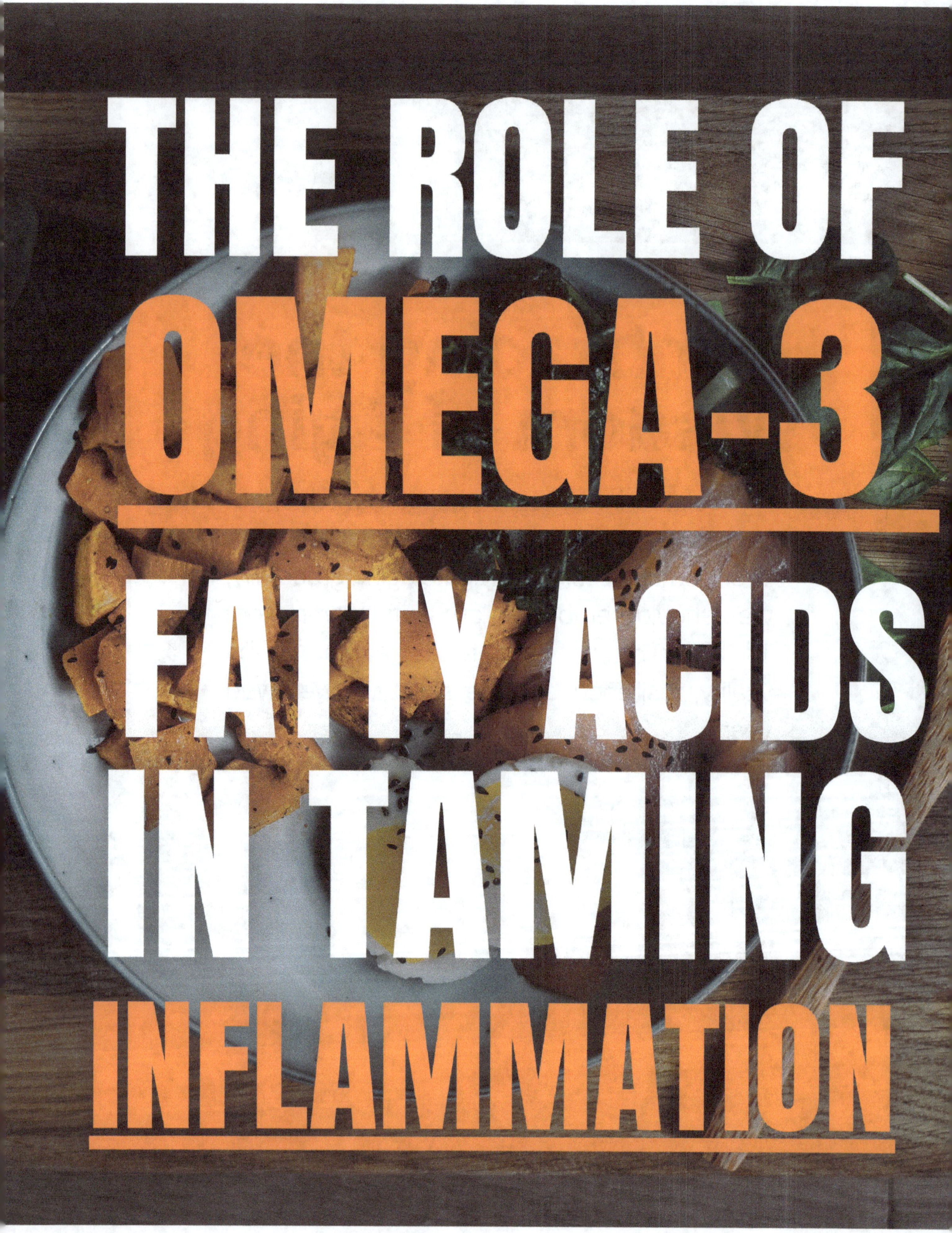

THE ROLE OF OMEGA-3 FATTY ACIDS IN TAMING INFLAMMATION

THEY HAVE REMARKABLE ANTI-INFLAMMATORY PROPERTIES AND ARE ABUNDANT IN CERTAIN FOODS AND SUPPLEMENTS.

Omega-3 fatty acids are allies in the fight against inflammation. They have an intricate tapestry that we will explore.

Understanding Omega-3 Fatty Acids: The Good Fats

Omega-3 fatty acids are essential for the body's proper functioning. They are a group of polyunsaturated fats that play pivotal roles in cellular function, brain health, and inflammation regulation. The three primary types of omega-3 fatty acids are alpha-linolenic acid (ALA), eicosapentaenoic acid (EPA), and docosahexaenoic acid (DHA).

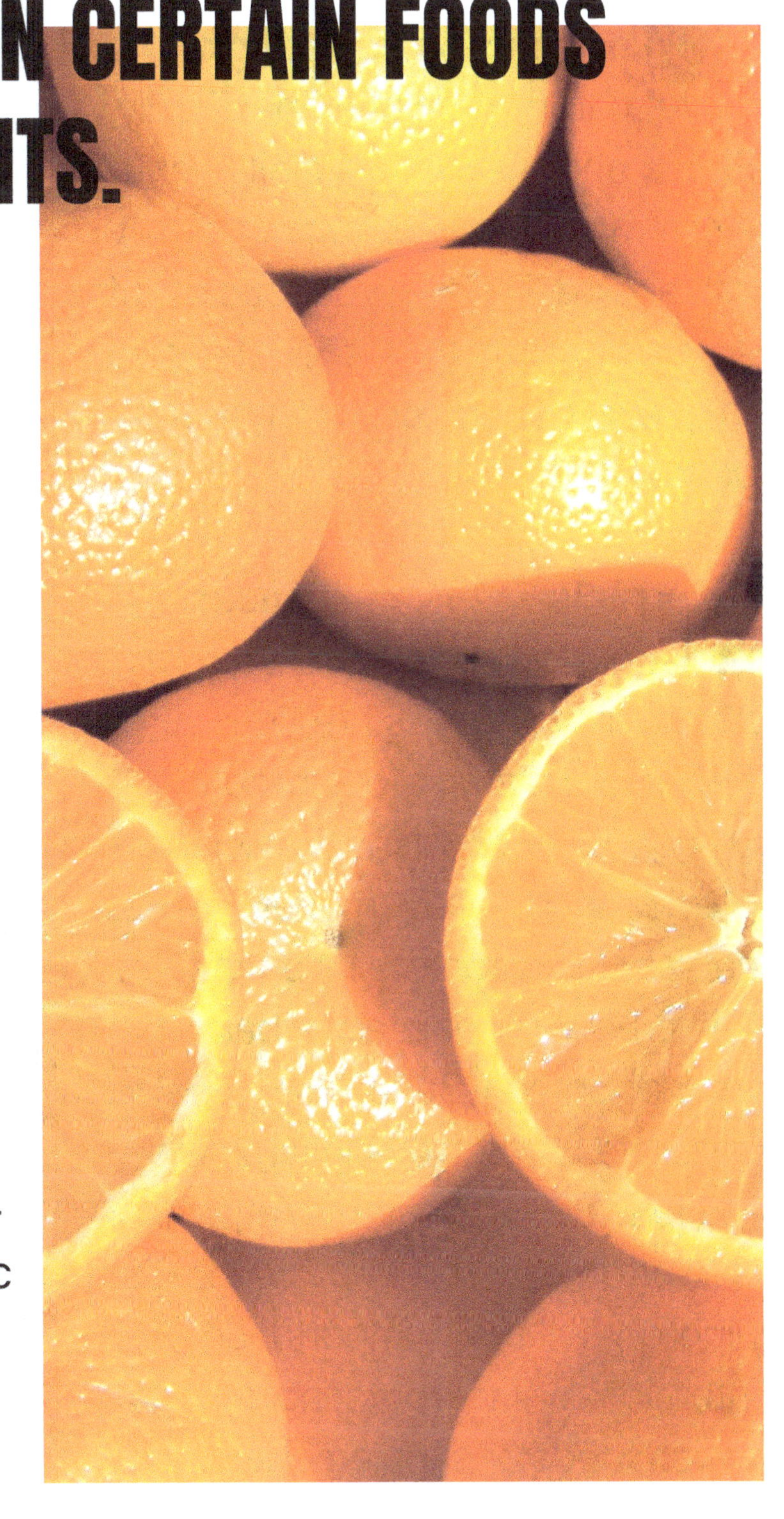

THE INFLAMMATION CONNECTION: OMEGA-3S AS NATURAL MODULATORS

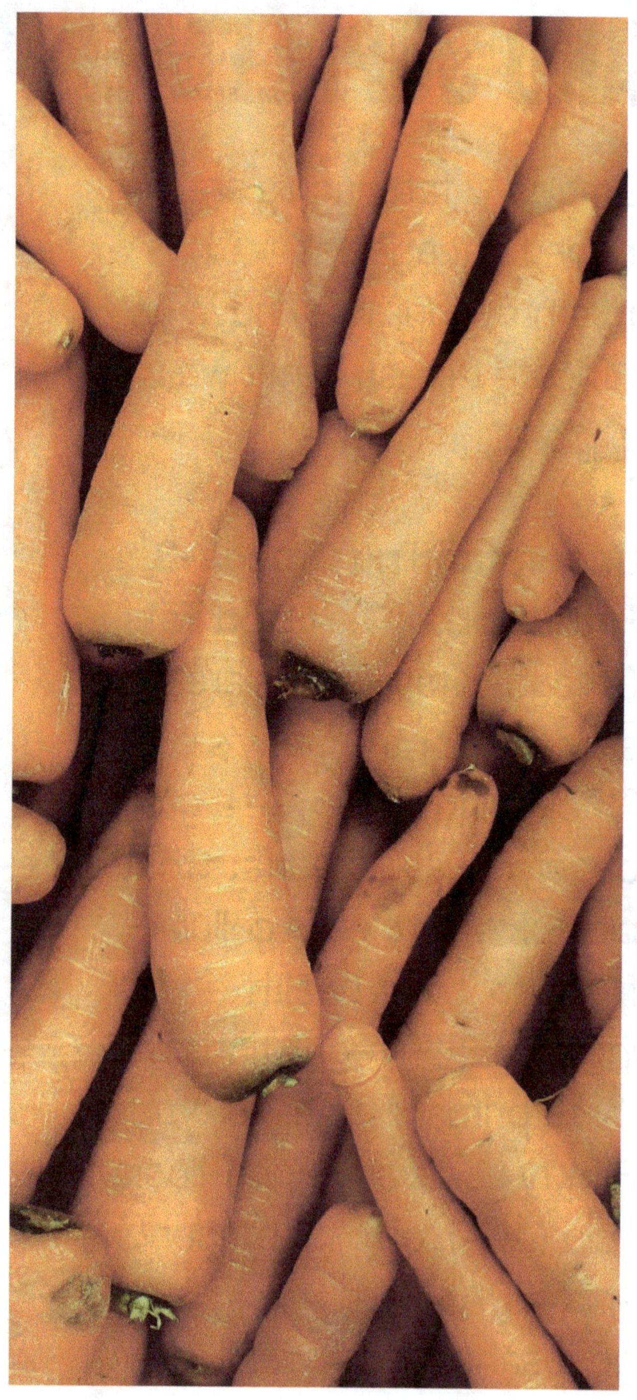

Inflammation is a natural and necessary response, but it can become problematic when it persists or becomes chronic. Omega-3 fatty acids can help by acting as natural modulators of the inflammatory process. Specifically, EPA and DHA exhibit anti-inflammatory effects by influencing the production of signaling molecules and reducing the expression of inflammatory genes.

Omega-3s vs. Omega-6s: Striking a Balance

Although omega-3s are known for their anti-inflammatory properties, omega-6 fatty acids, which are prevalent in many modern diets, can actually promote inflammation. It is crucial to maintain a balanced ratio of omega-3s to omega-6s to ensure a harmonious inflammatory response. The Western diet, which is often rich in omega-6s, highlights the importance of intentionally incorporating omega-3-rich foods or supplements.

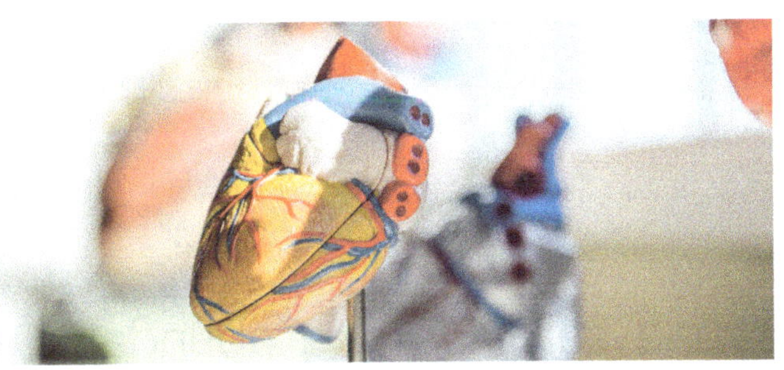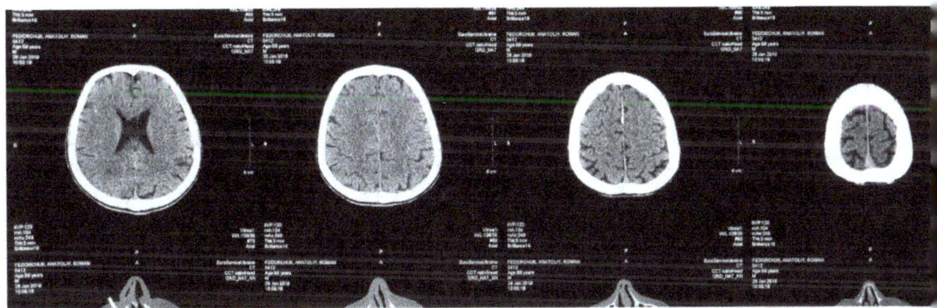

HEART HEALTH AND OMEGA-3S: A CARDIOVASCULAR SYMPHONY

Omega-3 fatty acids have been extensively studied for their cardiovascular benefits. They contribute to heart health by reducing blood clotting, lowering blood pressure, and improving overall vascular function. Regular consumption of omega-3-rich foods or supplements has been associated with a decreased risk of cardiovascular diseases, making them a cornerstone of heart-healthy nutrition.

OMEGA-3S AND BRAIN FUNCTION: NOURISHING THE MIND

DHA is a type of omega-3 fatty acid that is a major component of the brain. It has been linked to cognitive function and mental health. Adequate intake of omega-3s is associated with a lower risk of age-related cognitive decline and neurodegenerative conditions. Incorporating omega-3s into the diet is a proactive strategy for nurturing brain health and supporting cognitive well-being.

INFLAMMATION IN THE JOINTS: OMEGA-3S AS JOINT GUARDIANS

Omega-3 fatty acids may help alleviate joint pain and stiffness by exhibiting anti-inflammatory effects. Including omega-3-rich foods or supplements can be a valuable component of a holistic approach to joint health.

NATURAL SOURCES OF OMEGA-3S: FROM SEA TO TABLE

Certain fish, such as salmon, mackerel, and sardines, are abundant sources of omega-3 fatty acids. Plant-based sources, such as flaxseeds, chia seeds, and walnuts, provide ALA. Although these foods offer valuable omega-3s, some individuals may prefer fish oil supplements or algae-based supplements, especially for DHA and EPA, to ensure a consistent and concentrated intake.

NAVIGATING OMEGA-3 SUPPLEMENTATION: A PERSONALIZED APPROACH

To optimize your omega-3 intake, consider supplementing with fish oil capsules or algae-based supplements. These provide a concentrated source of EPA and DHA. It's important to consult with a healthcare professional before incorporating supplements, taking into account factors such as dietary habits, health conditions, and potential interactions.

POTENTIAL RISKS AND CONSIDERATIONS: A BALANCED PERSPECTIVE

Although omega-3 fatty acids offer many health benefits, it is important to consume them in moderation. Excessive intake, whether through supplements or specific foods, may have potential risks, such as an increased risk of bleeding. To navigate the nuanced terrain of omega-3 supplementation, it is important to strike a balance and seek guidance from healthcare professionals.

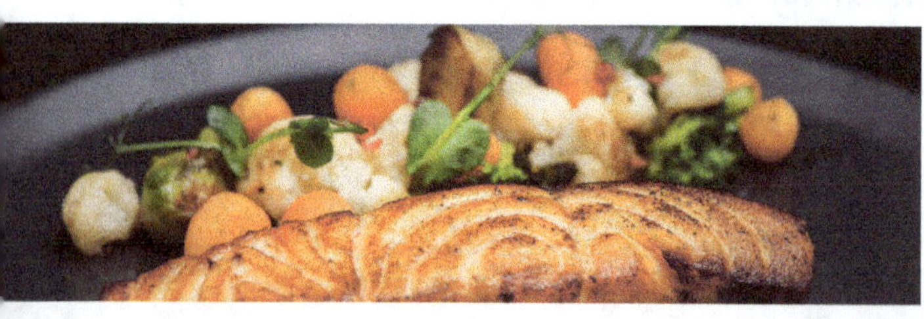
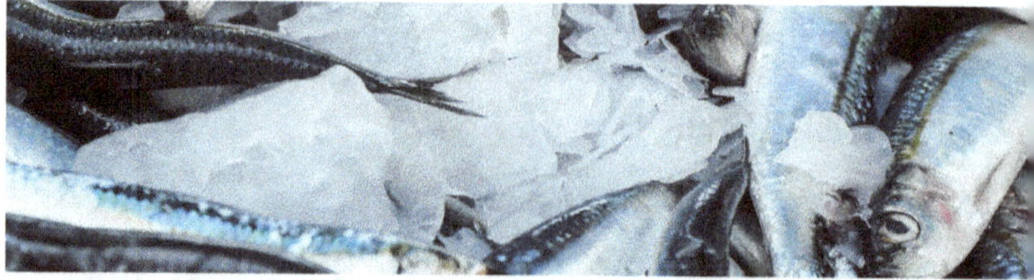

HARNESSING THE HEALING POTENTIAL OF OMEGA-3S

In the quest for holistic well-being, omega-3 fatty acids are emerging as powerful allies in the ongoing battle against inflammation. From cardiovascular health to joint support and cognitive function, the benefits of these essential fats extend to various facets of our health. Whether through judicious food choices or supplementation, integrating omega-3s into our lifestyle becomes a proactive step towards nourishing our bodies and taming the flames of inflammation - a journey towards optimal health and vitality.

PART 2

EAT SMARTER FOR A HEALTHIER YOU

To achieve optimal health, we must carefully choose the foods we eat every day. These choices have a significant impact on the inflammation balance in our bodies. An anti-inflammatory plate requires a deliberate selection of foods that not only taste good but also work together to reduce inflammation. In this text, we will explore how to create a plate that promotes well-being and vitality.

Leafy Greens as Cornerstones

Dark, leafy greens like kale, spinach, and Swiss chard are nutritional powerhouses that deserve a prominent place on your plate. Packed with vitamins, minerals, and antioxidants, these greens offer a myriad of health benefits, including anti-inflammatory properties.

Foundations of Color and Diversity

A diverse range of colorful foods can be seen on a vibrant plate. Fruits and vegetables of various hues are rich in antioxidants, vitamins, and minerals. These plant-based powerhouses not only provide essential nutrients but also contribute to a well-rounded and inflammation-fighting diet.

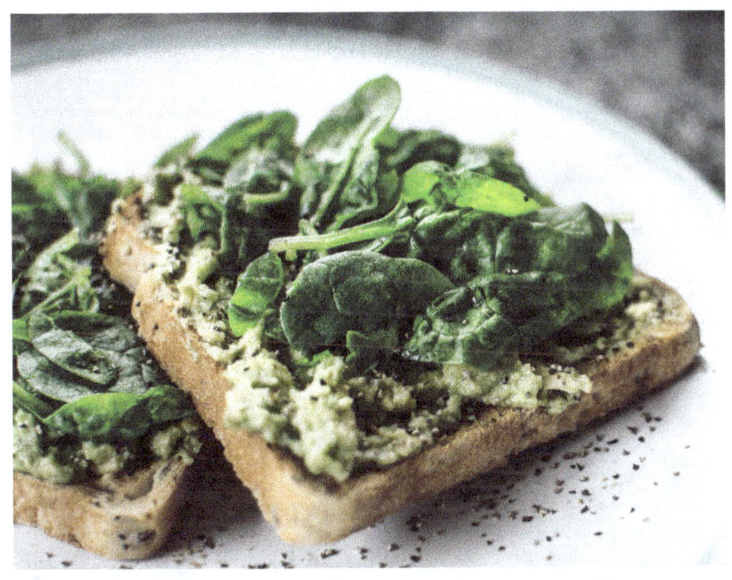

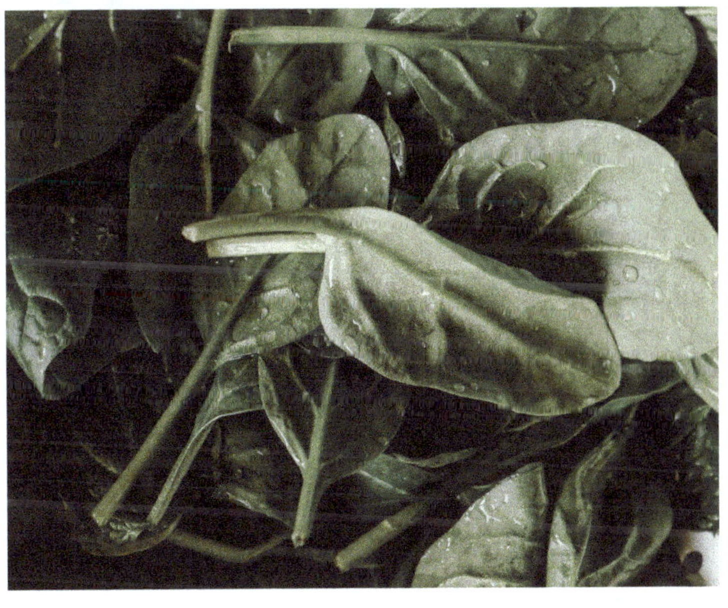

WHOLE GRAINS FOR SUSTAINED ENERGY

Incorporating whole grains, such as quinoa, brown rice, and oats, adds a wholesome dimension to your anti-inflammatory plate. Whole grains are rich in fiber and nutrients, providing sustained energy and contributing to a balanced inflammatory response.

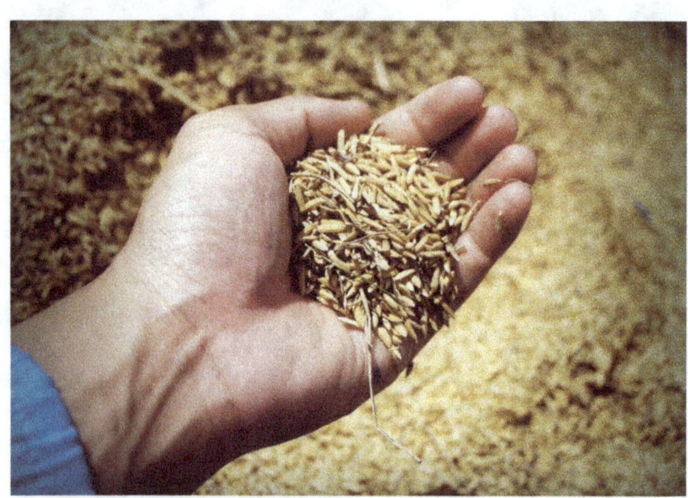

LEAN PROTEINS FOR MUSCLE SUPPORT

Choose lean protein sources such as poultry, tofu, or legumes to promote muscle health. Protein is necessary for tissue repair and immune function, which helps create an overall anti-inflammatory environment.

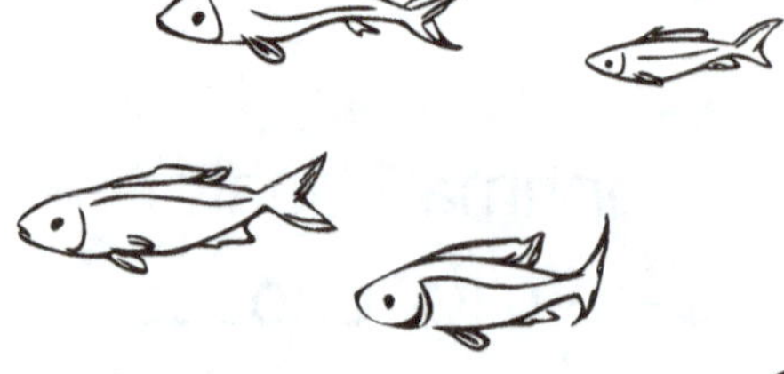

OMEGA-3 RICH FATTY FISH

Fatty fish, such as salmon, mackerel, and sardines, provide a potent dose of omega-3 fatty acids. These essential fats play a crucial role in reducing inflammation and supporting overall cardiovascular health. It is recommended to include these types of fish in your diet.

HEALTHY FATS FROM AVOCADO AND NUTS

Incorporate healthy fat sources like avocados, almonds, and walnuts. These foods provide monounsaturated fats and antioxidants, which help balance inflammation and promote heart health.

BERRIES FOR ANTIOXIDANT BOOSTS

Berries, such as blueberries, strawberries, and raspberries, are rich in antioxidants. They can help fight oxidative stress and inflammation in the body.

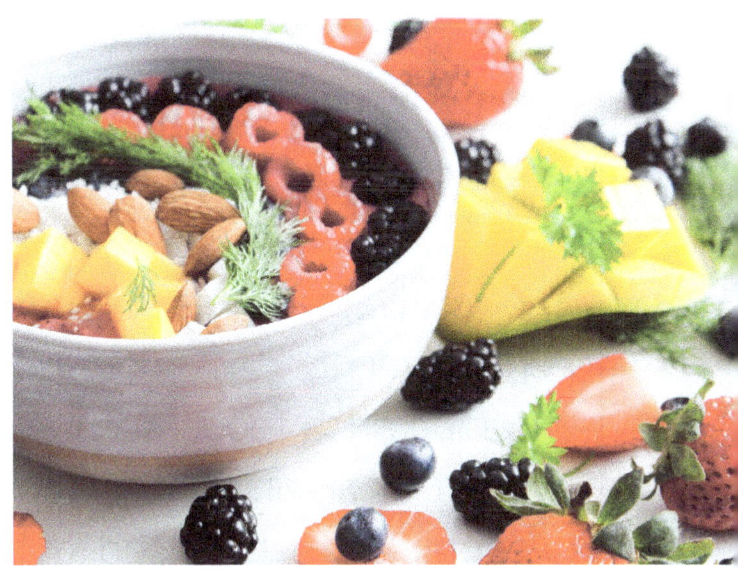

HERBS AND SPICES AS FLAVORFUL ALLIES

Embrace the rich flavors of herbs and spices while benefiting from their anti-inflammatory properties. Turmeric, ginger, garlic, and cinnamon add zest to your dishes and actively reduce inflammation within the body.

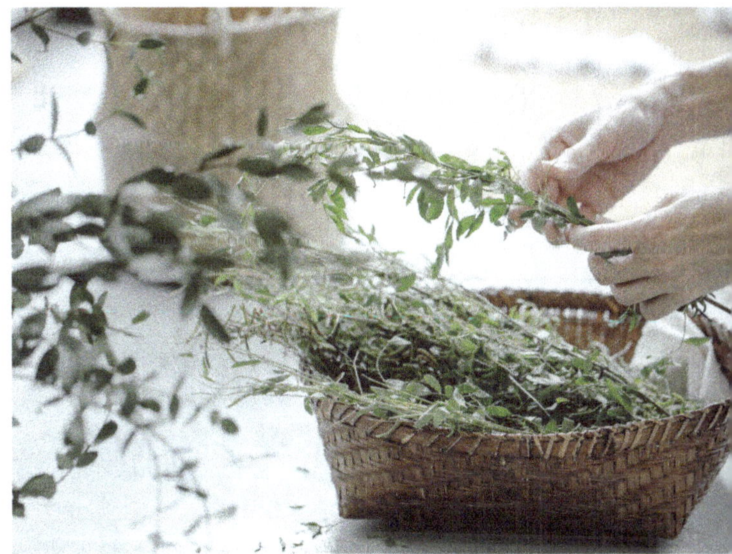

PROBIOTIC-RICH FOODS FOR GUT HEALTH

To cultivate a healthy gut environment, include probiotic-rich foods such as yogurt, kefir, and fermented vegetables. A balanced gut microbiome is associated with reduced inflammation and improved overall well-being.

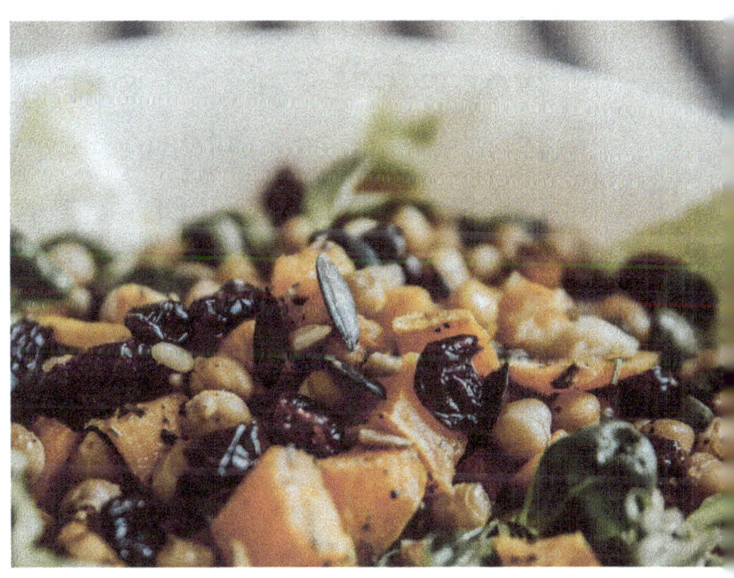

HYDRATION WITH GREEN TEA

To cultivate a healthy gut environment, include probiotic-rich foods such as yogurt, kefir, and fermented vegetables. A balanced gut microbiome is associated with reduced inflammation and improved overall well-being.

MINDFUL EATING PRACTICES

To build an anti-inflammatory plate, it is important to do more than just select the right foods. You should also incorporate mindful eating practices, such as savoring each bite, chewing thoroughly, and being attuned to hunger and fullness cues.

LIMITING PROCESSED AND SUGARY FOODS

To build an anti-inflammatory plate, minimize processed and sugary foods. These items can cause inflammation and disrupt the delicate balance of an anti-inflammatory diet.

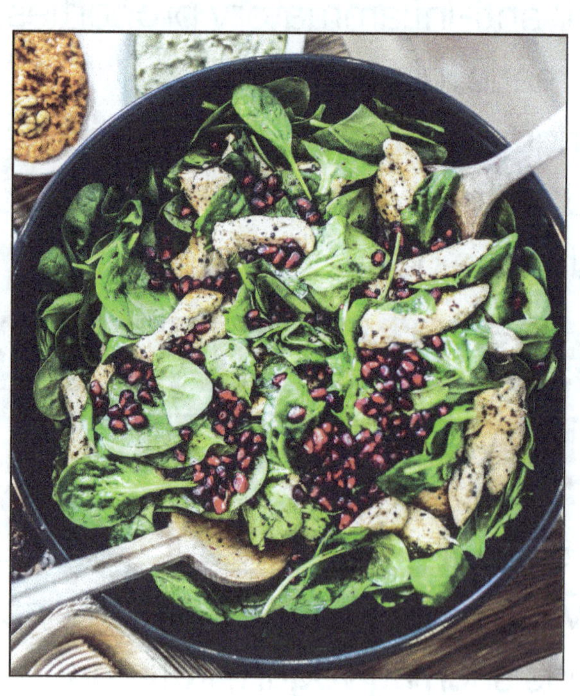

A SYMPHONY OF WELLNESS ON YOUR PLATE

Crafting an anti-inflammatory plate is easy and delicious. By incorporating a variety of nutrient-rich whole foods into a balanced and colorful meal, you can improve your overall well-being. Use simple, flavorful ingredients to create a culinary journey that not only delights your palate but also promotes vitality and wellness.

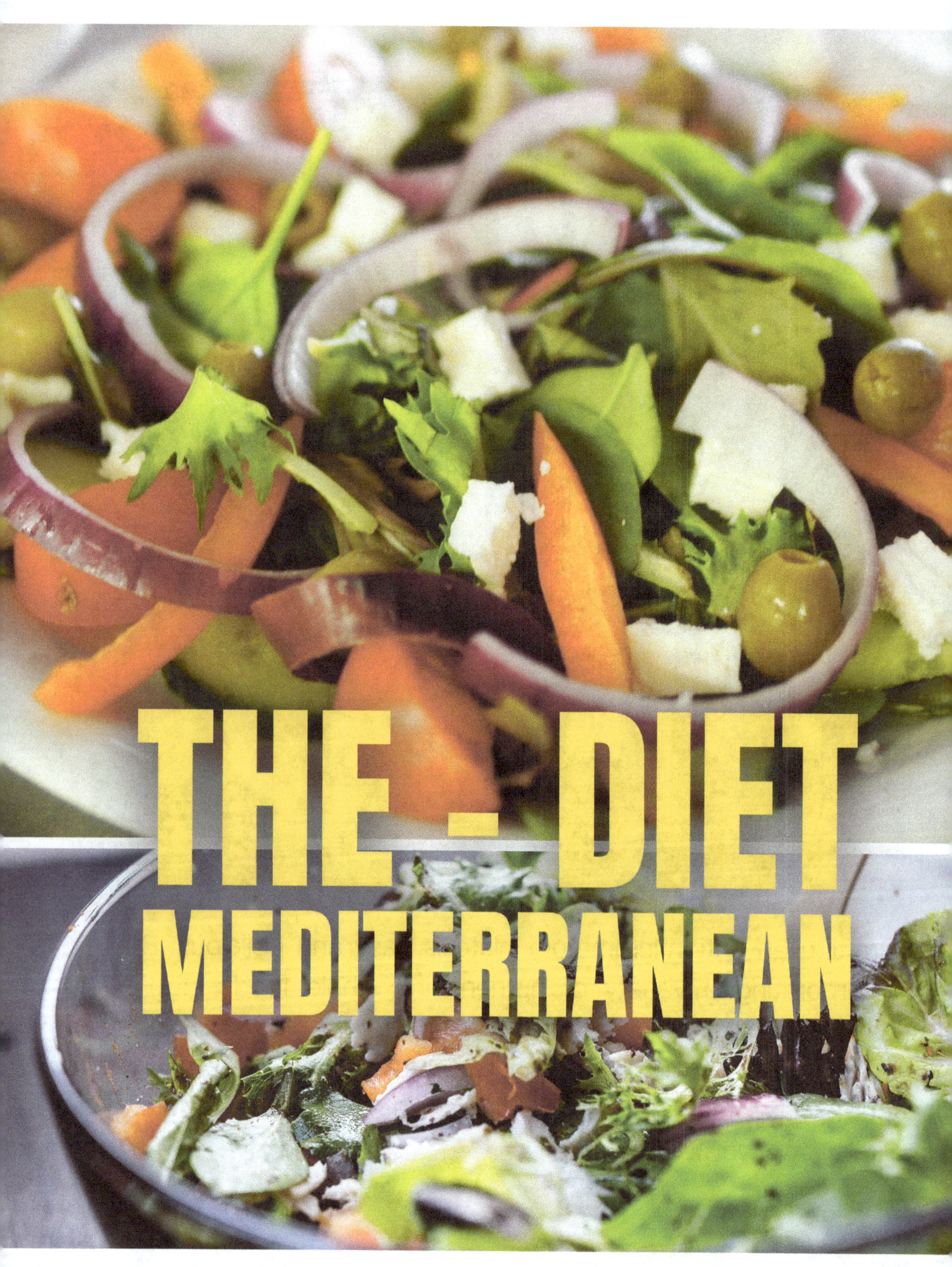
THE - DIET
MEDITERRANEAN

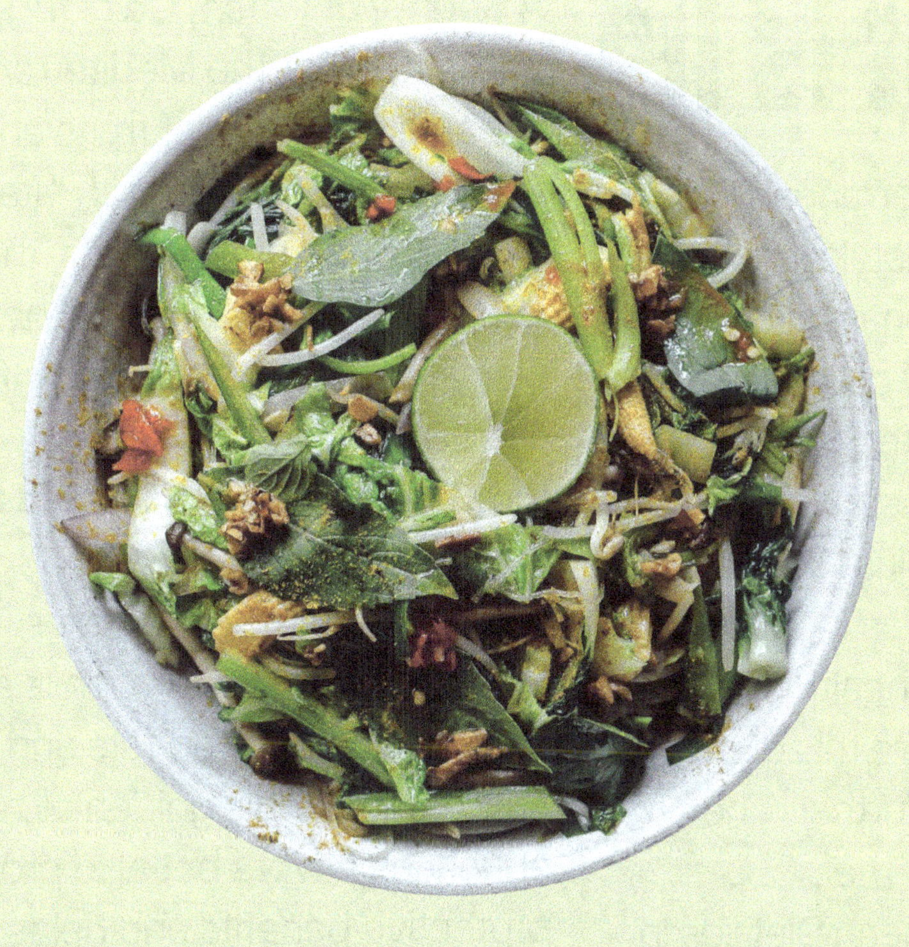

FLAVORFUL APPROACH TO INFLAMMATION CONTROL

What is it?

The Mediterranean Diet is a healthy lifestyle inspired by the traditional eating patterns of countries bordering the Mediterranean Sea. It is more than just a collection of recipes, as it offers numerous health benefits. Let's explore this dietary approach further. The essence of the Mediterranean Diet lies in its rich tapestry of flavors, nutrients, and well-being woven into its culinary philosophy.

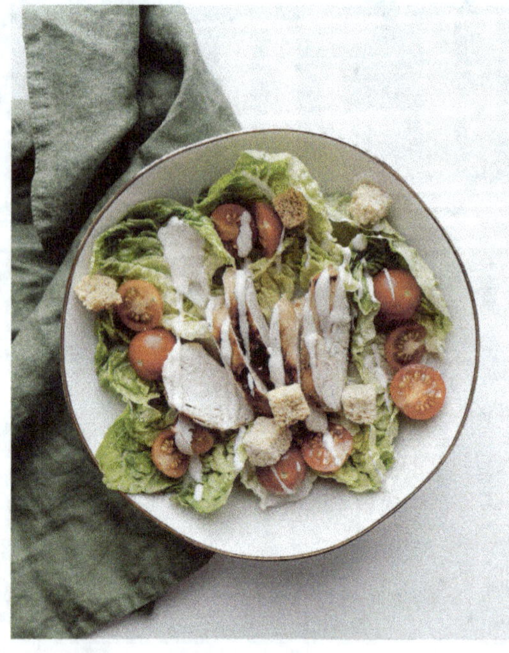

A Bounty of Fresh, Colorful Produce

At the heart of the Mediterranean Diet lies an abundance of fruits and vegetables. Bursting with vitamins, minerals, and antioxidants, these colorful gems contribute to overall health and play a vital role in reducing inflammation

Extra Virgin Olive Oil: Liquid Gold for Hea

Mediterranean cuisine relies heavily on extra virgin olive oil, which is a rich source of monounsaturated fats and antioxidants. This golden oil not only enhances flavors but also provides heart-protective benefits and helps maintain a balanced inflammatory response.

Whole Grains for Sustained Energy

The Mediterranean Diet emphasizes the consumption of whole grains such as farro, bulgur, and whole wheat bread. The diet's focus on whole grains makes it an excellent choice for those looking to improve their overall health. These grains provide complex carbohydrates, fiber, and a range of nutrients, which support sustained energy levels and promote a healthy gut.

Lean Proteins: A Balanced Approach

The Mediterranean Diet emphasizes lean protein sources such as fish, poultry, beans, and legumes. Red meat should be consumed in moderation. These foods provide essential amino acids, promote muscle health, and contribute to an overall anti-inflammatory environment.

Fruits of the Sea: Omega-3 Richness

Fatty fish such as salmon, mackerel, and sardines make frequent appearances in Mediterranean dishes. These oceanic delights bring a hearty dose of omega-3 fatty acids, supporting heart health and actively reducing inflammation.

Nuts and Seeds for Crunch and Nutrients

Almonds, walnuts, and sunflower seeds are nutrient-packed snacks or meal additions. They are rich in healthy fats, fiber, and a spectrum of vitamins and minerals, contributing to overall well-being.

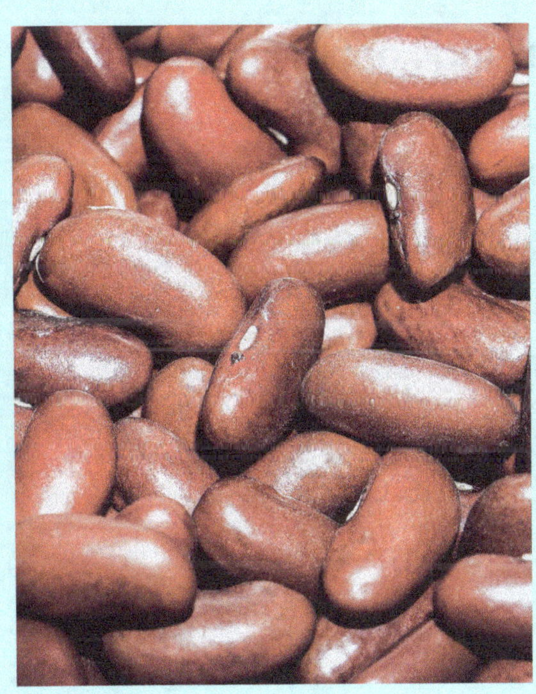
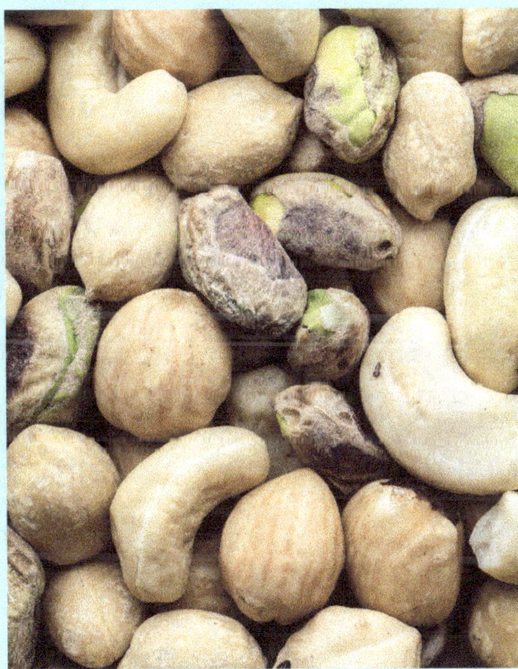
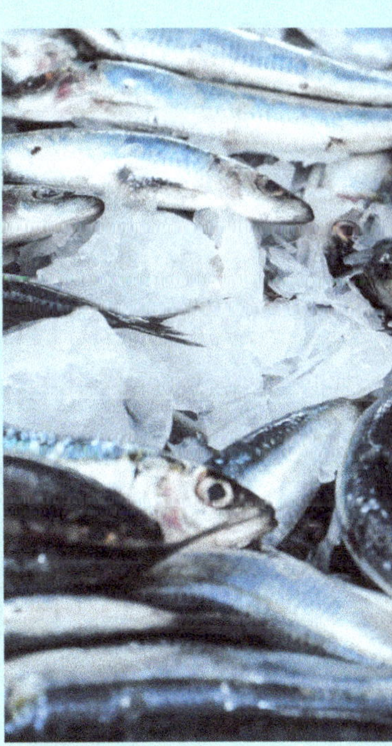

Dairy in Moderation

The Mediterranean Diet includes dairy products like cheese and yogurt, which should be consumed in moderation. These foods provide calcium and probiotics, adding a creamy texture to meals while also promoting bone health and gut microbiome balance.

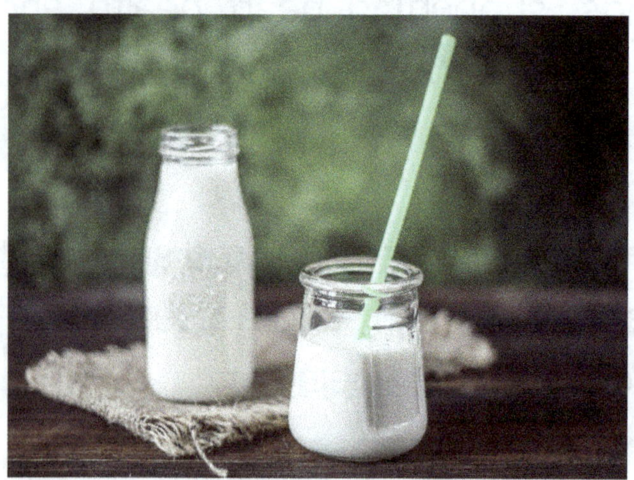

Wine in Moderation: A Toast to Longevity

The Mediterranean Diet involves moderate consumption of red wine with meals. Red wine is rich in antioxidants and associated with heart health and longevity, adding a convivial touch to the dining experience.

Herbs and Spices: Flavorful Medicine

Basil, oregano, garlic, and rosemary are herbs and spices that are essential to the Mediterranean Diet. They not only enhance the taste but also provide anti-inflammatory properties, contributing to the diet's overall health benefits.

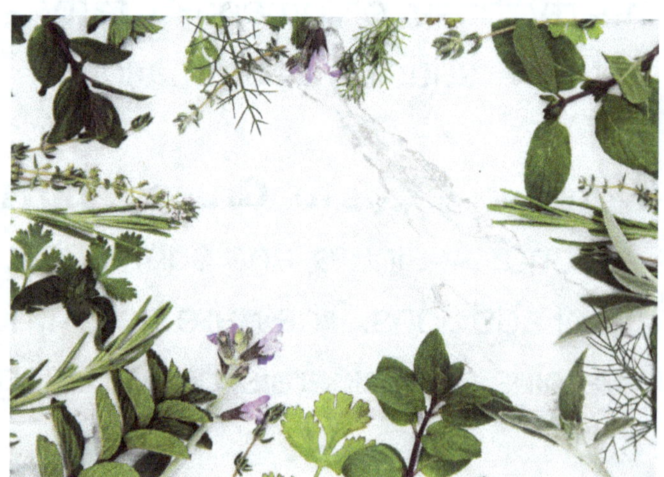

Seasonal and Local: Harmony with Nature

The "diet" promotes the use of locally sourced and seasonal ingredients. This supports environmental sustainability and ensures the freshness and nutritional value of the food consumed.

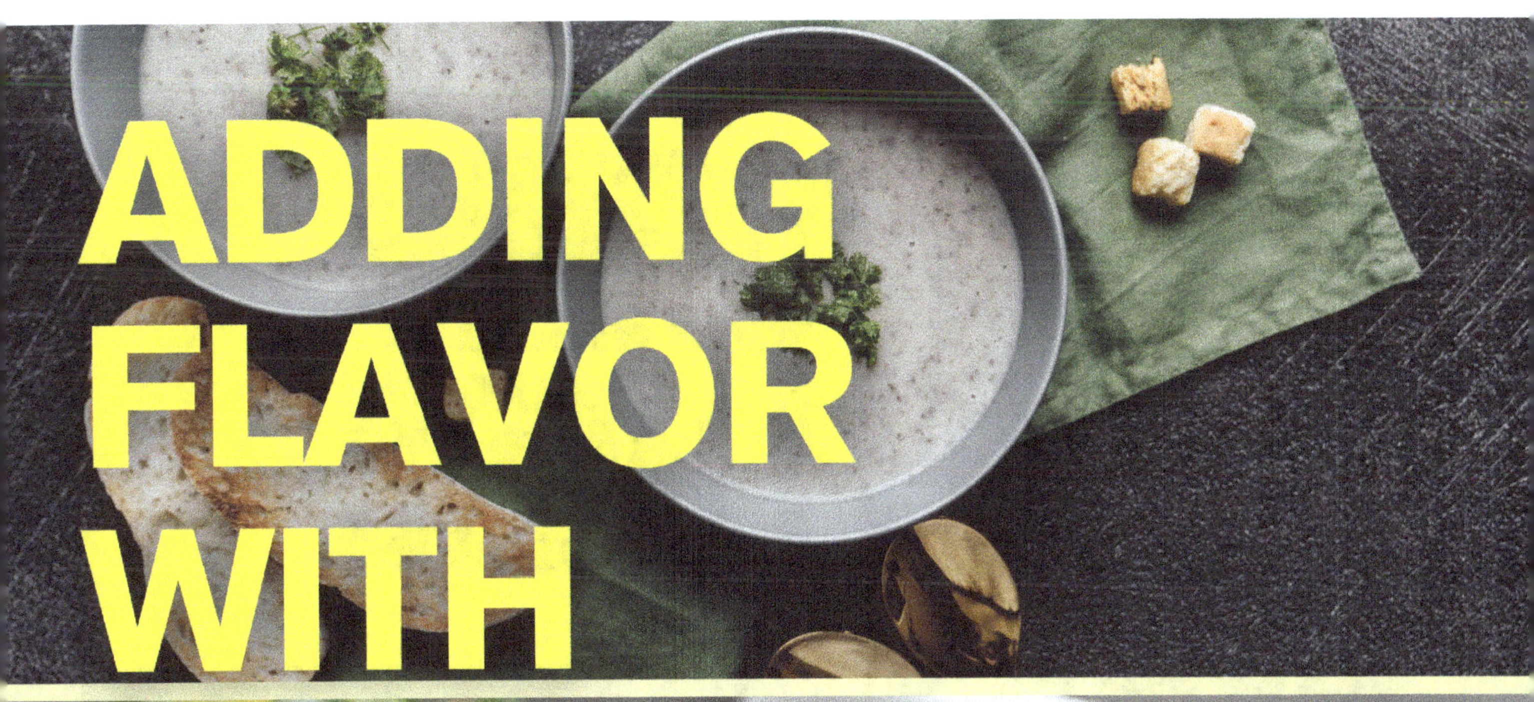

ADDING FLAVOR WITH

ANTI-INFLAMMATORY PUNCH

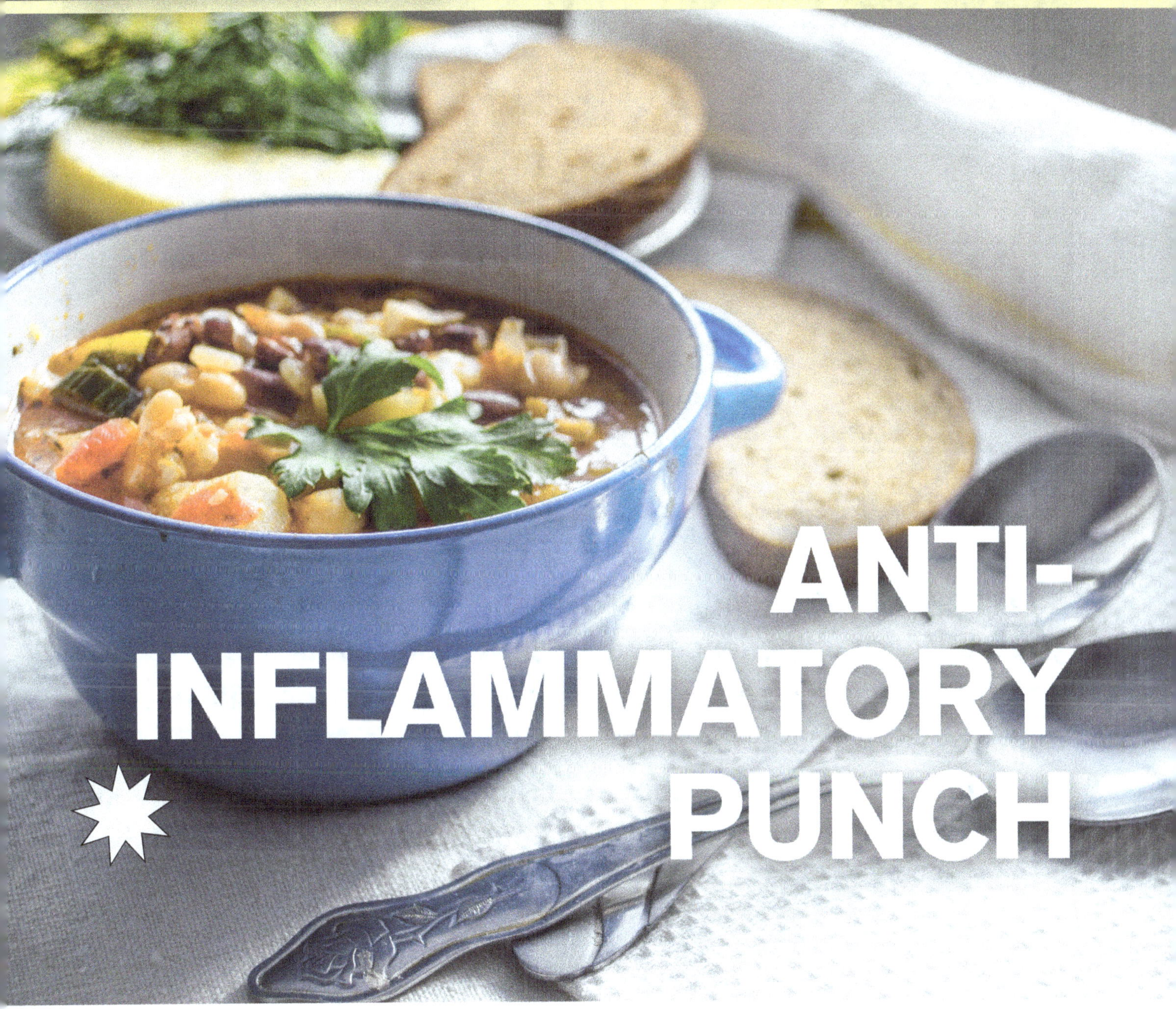

SAVORING WELLNESS

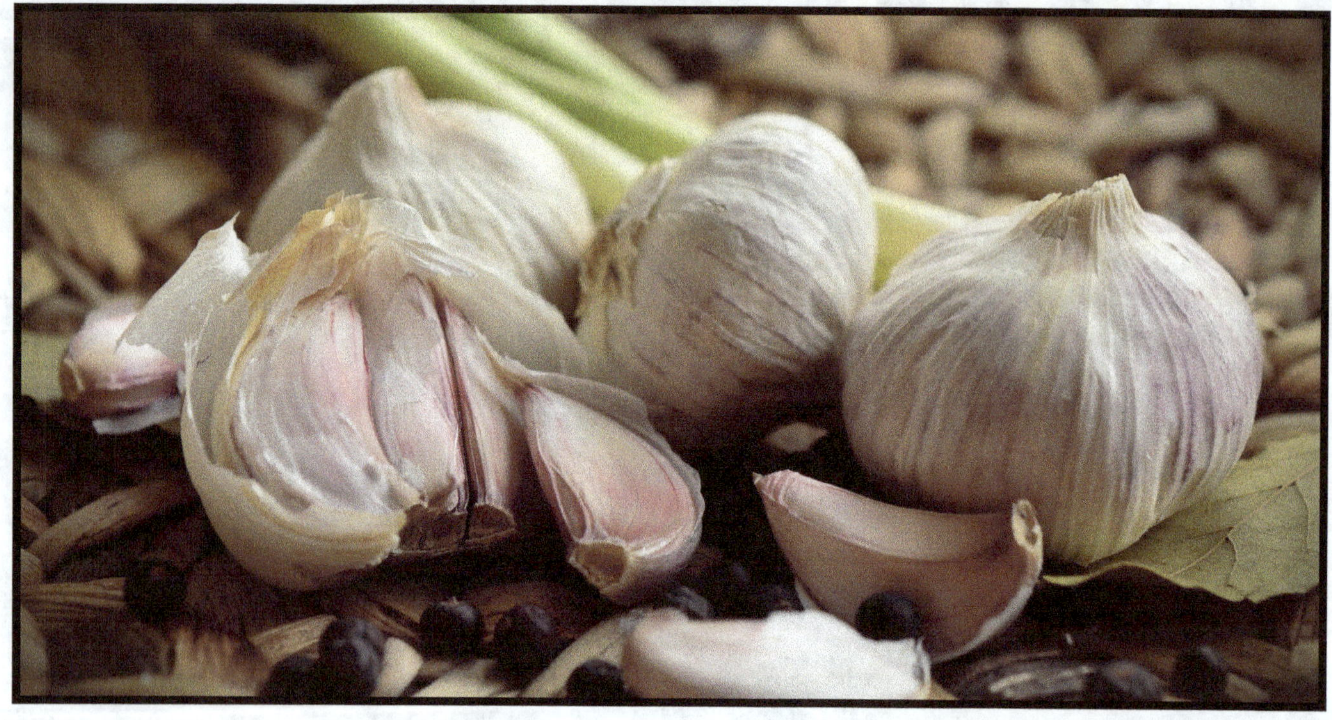

Infusing your meals with an anti-inflammatory punch can elevate your culinary experience while prioritizing your health. This approach to cooking embraces a symphony of flavors that not only tantalizes the taste buds but also actively contributes to reducing inflammation within the body. Let's delve into the art of adding vibrant, anti-inflammatory flair to your dishes, turning every bite into a celebration of well-being.

GINGER: ZEST FOR LIFE

Unleash the zesty goodness of ginger in your culinary creations. With its anti-inflammatory and antioxidant properties, ginger lends a refreshing kick to both savory and sweet dishes. Grate it into stir-fries, brew it into tea, or incorporate it into marinades for a burst of vibrant flavor

GARLIC: NATURE'S FLAVOR BOOSTER

Garlic is a versatile ingredient that is celebrated for its culinary charm and health benefits. It is rich in allicin, which offers anti-inflammatory and immune-boosting effects. You can roast it, sauté it, or incorporate it into dressings to elevate the flavor profile of your meals.

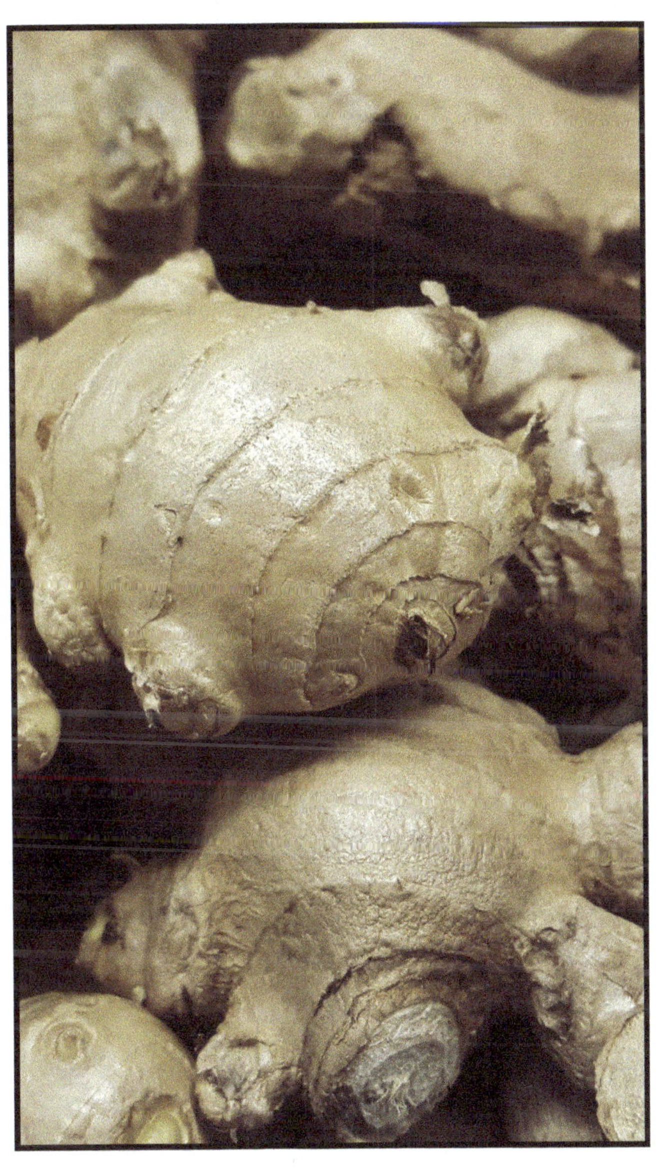

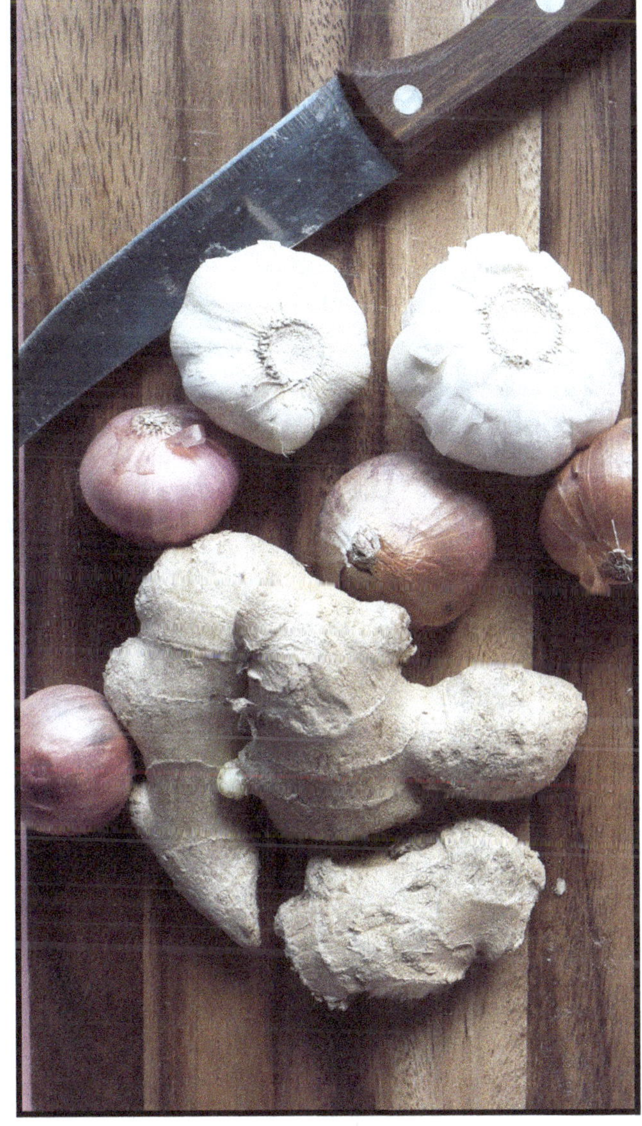

CINNAMON: SWEET AND SPICY HARMONY

Cinnamon has sweet and spicy notes and can be used in both sweet and savory dishes. Cinnamon has sweet and spicy notes and can be used in both sweet and savory dishes. Cinnamon has sweet and spicy notes and can be used in both sweet and savory dishes. It is also an anti-inflammatory spice that can add warmth to your meals. You can sprinkle it on oatmeal, incorporate it into savory stews, or infuse it into beverages to enliven your taste buds while promoting health.

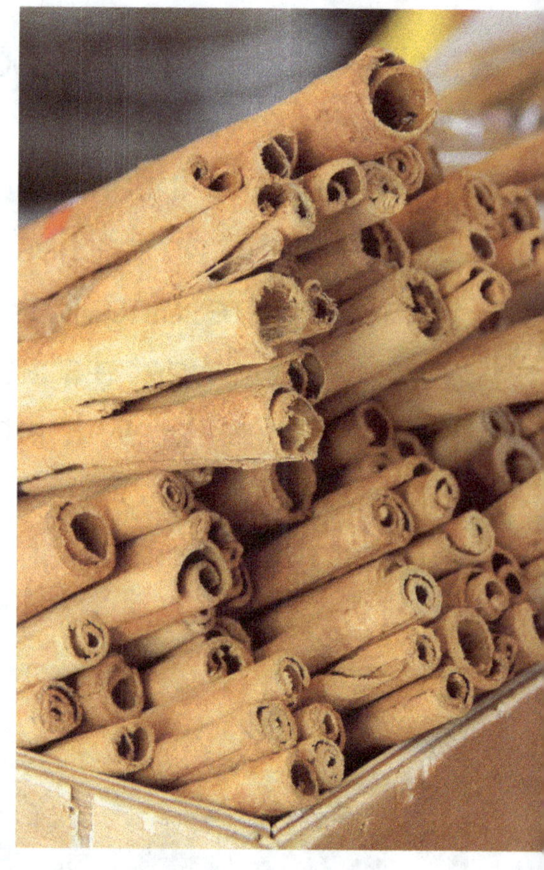

CITRUS ZEST AND JUICES

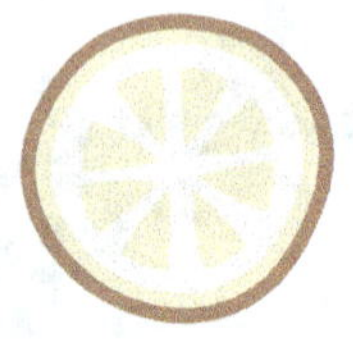
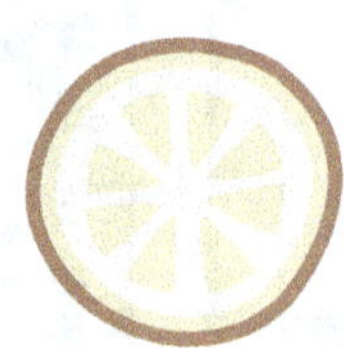

Citrus fruits, such as lemons, limes, and oranges, add tangy flavor to your meals. They are rich in vitamin C and antioxidants, which contribute to the anti-inflammatory profile of your culinary creations. You can use zest and juice to enhance the flavor of marinades, dressings, and desserts.

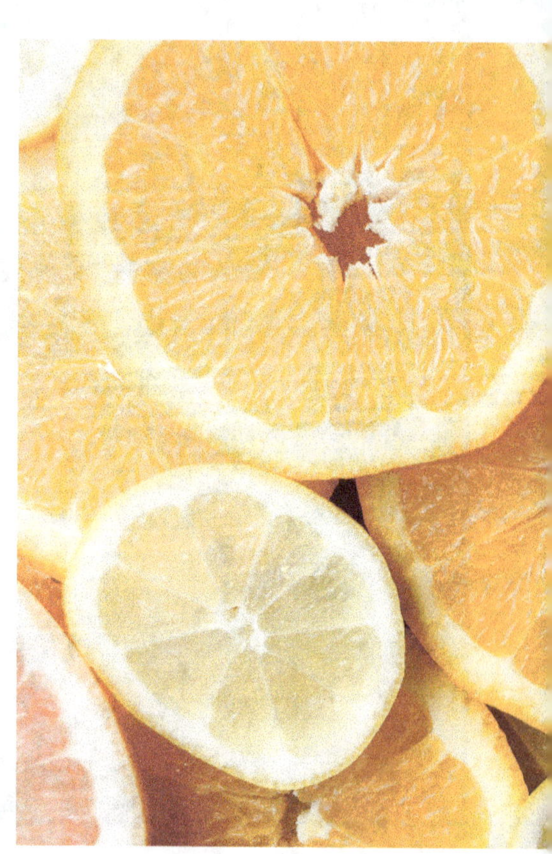

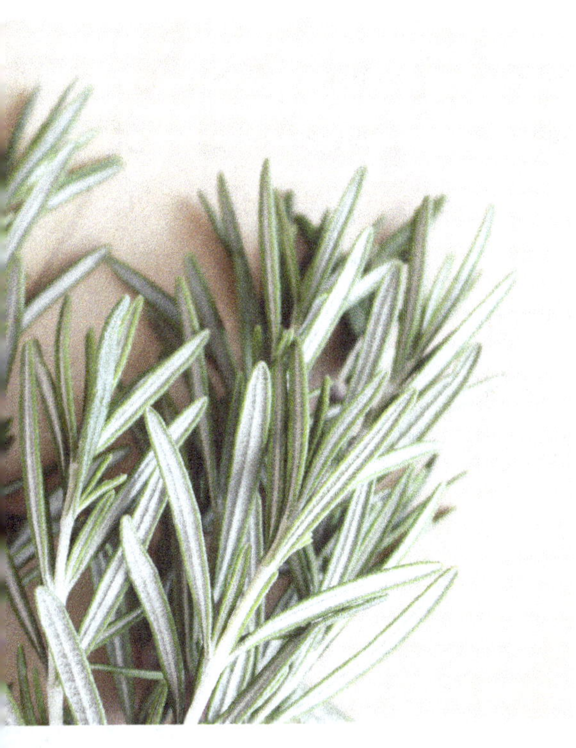

ROSEMARY: AROMATIC ELEGANCE

Enhance your dishes with the fragrant and sophisticated flavor of rosemary. In addition to its enticing aroma, rosemary contains anti-inflammatory compounds. You can roast vegetables with rosemary, add it to marinades, or use it as a flavorful garnish to create a culinary experience that delights the senses and promotes well-being.

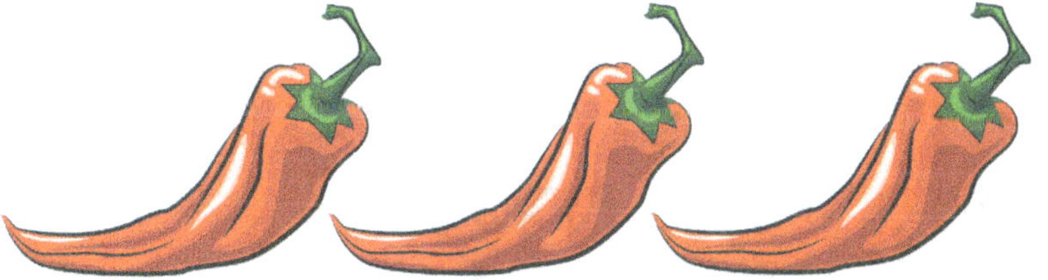

CHILI PEPPERS: SPICY HEAT WITH BENEFITS

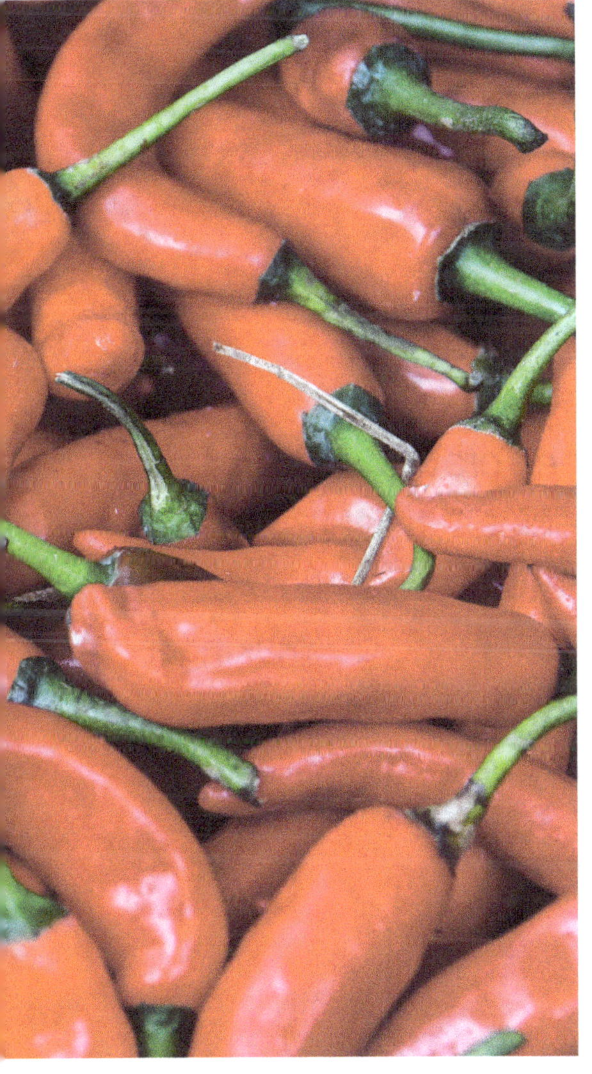

Chili peppers are known for their fiery flavor and anti-inflammatory properties due to capsaicin, the compound responsible for the heat. Capsaicin has been linked to reduced inflammation. Incorporate chili peppers into salsas, sauces, or spice blends for a bold and healthful culinary adventure.

ONIONS

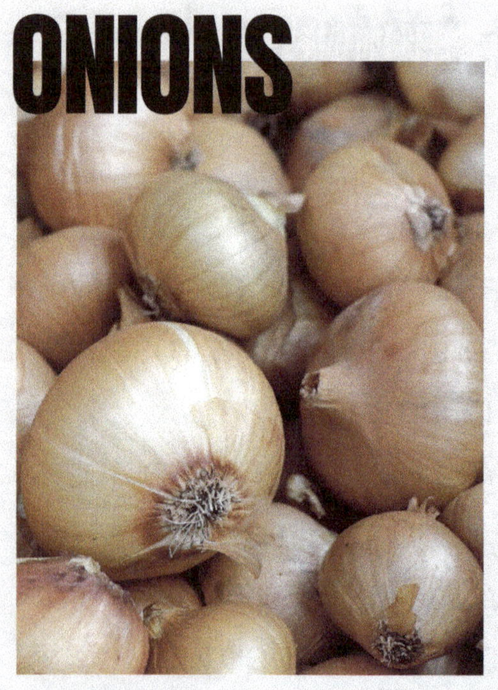

Enhance the flavor of your dishes by adding the savory sweetness of onions. Onions contain quercetin, an antioxidant that provides anti-inflammatory benefits. You can sauté, caramelize, or pickle onions to add depth and complexity to your meals.

DARK CHOCOLATE

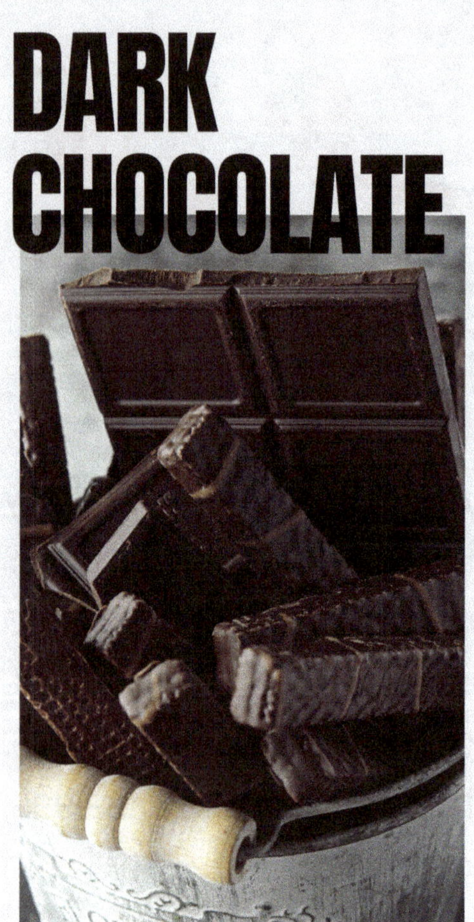

Satisfy your sweet cravings with dark chocolate, a delicious treat that also has anti-inflammatory properties. Dark chocolate is rich in flavonoids, making it a guilt-free addition to desserts or a satisfying and healthy sweet indulgence on its own.

KEEP IN MIND

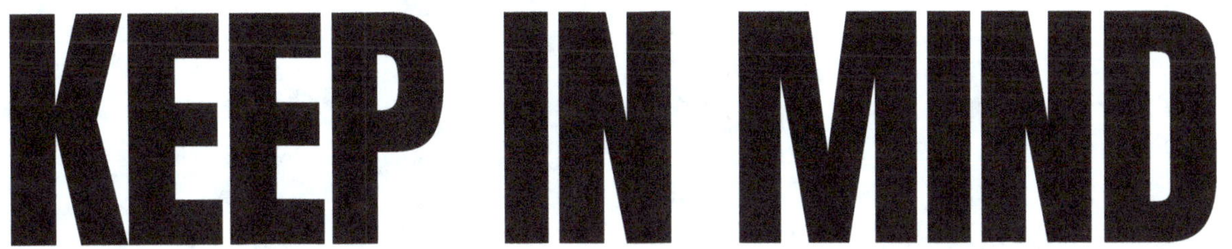

Adding anti-inflammatory ingredients to your meals is not only a culinary choice but also a celebration of vibrant flavors and well-being. By incorporating these health-enhancing ingredients into your cooking, you can elevate your gastronomic experience and contribute to a lifestyle that embraces the harmony of taste and vitality. Let every bite be a symphony of flavor, a toast to your health, and a culinary journey that celebrates the art of savoring wellness.

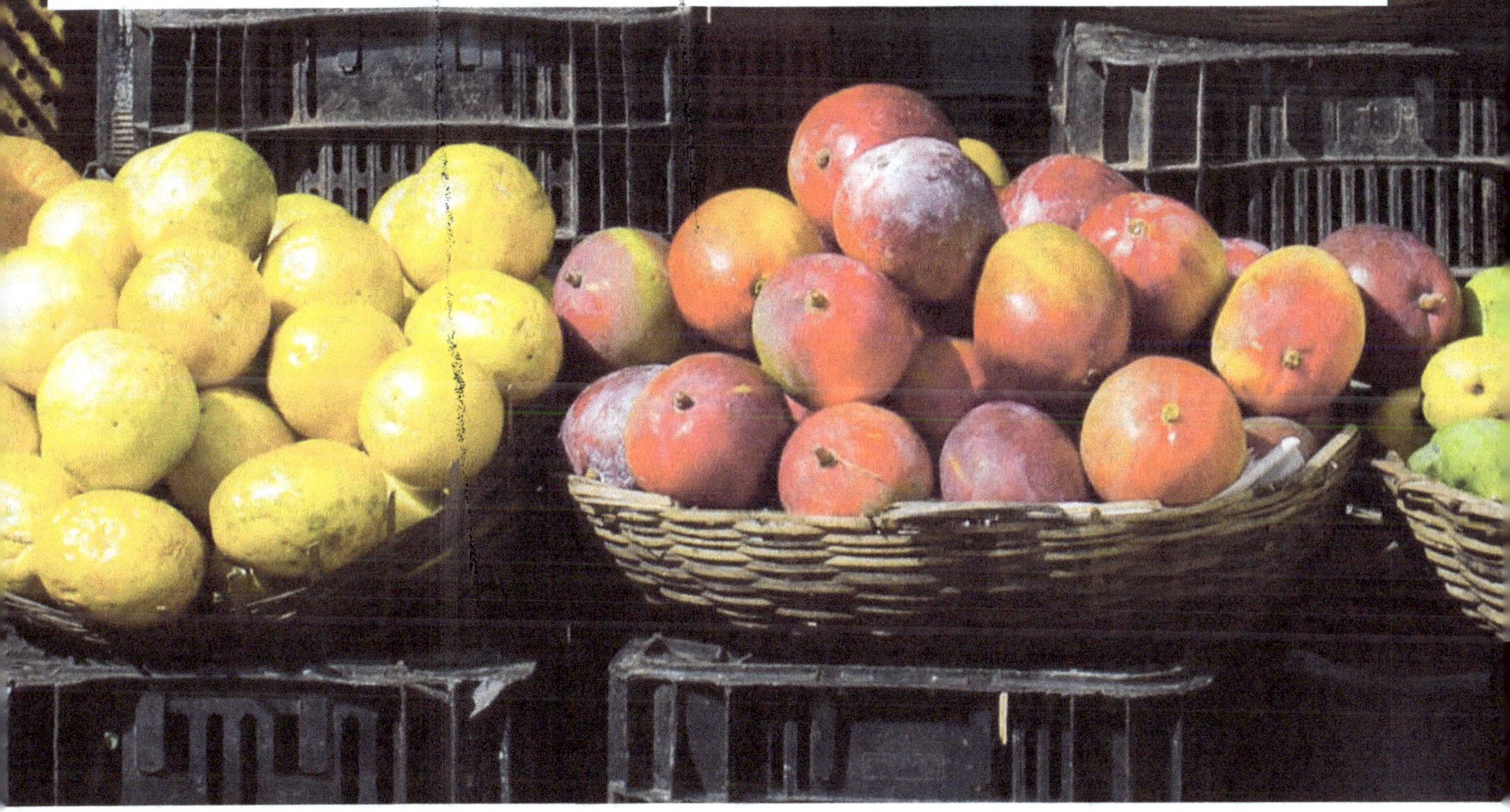

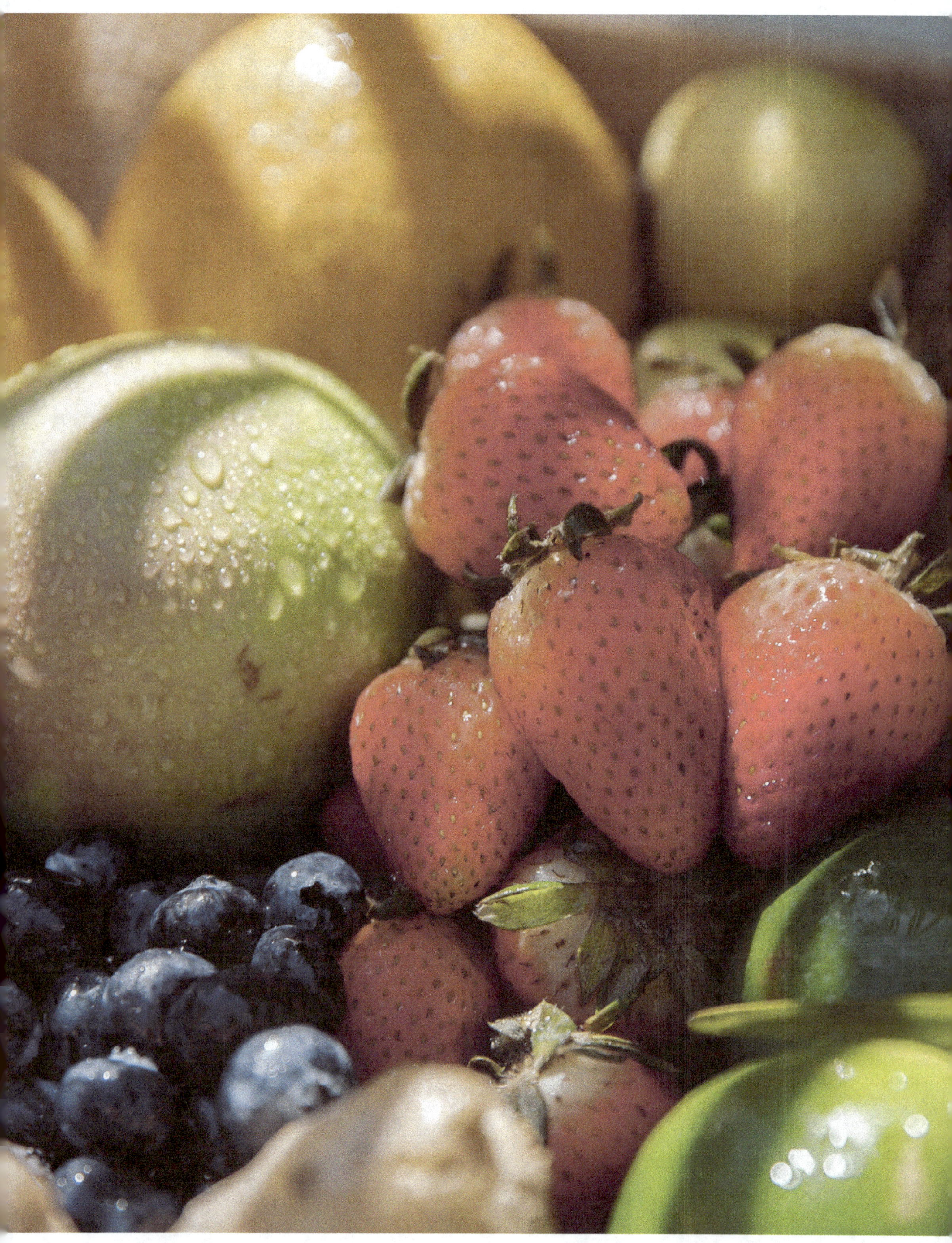

RELATIONSHIP BETWEEN SUGAR AND INFLAMMATION

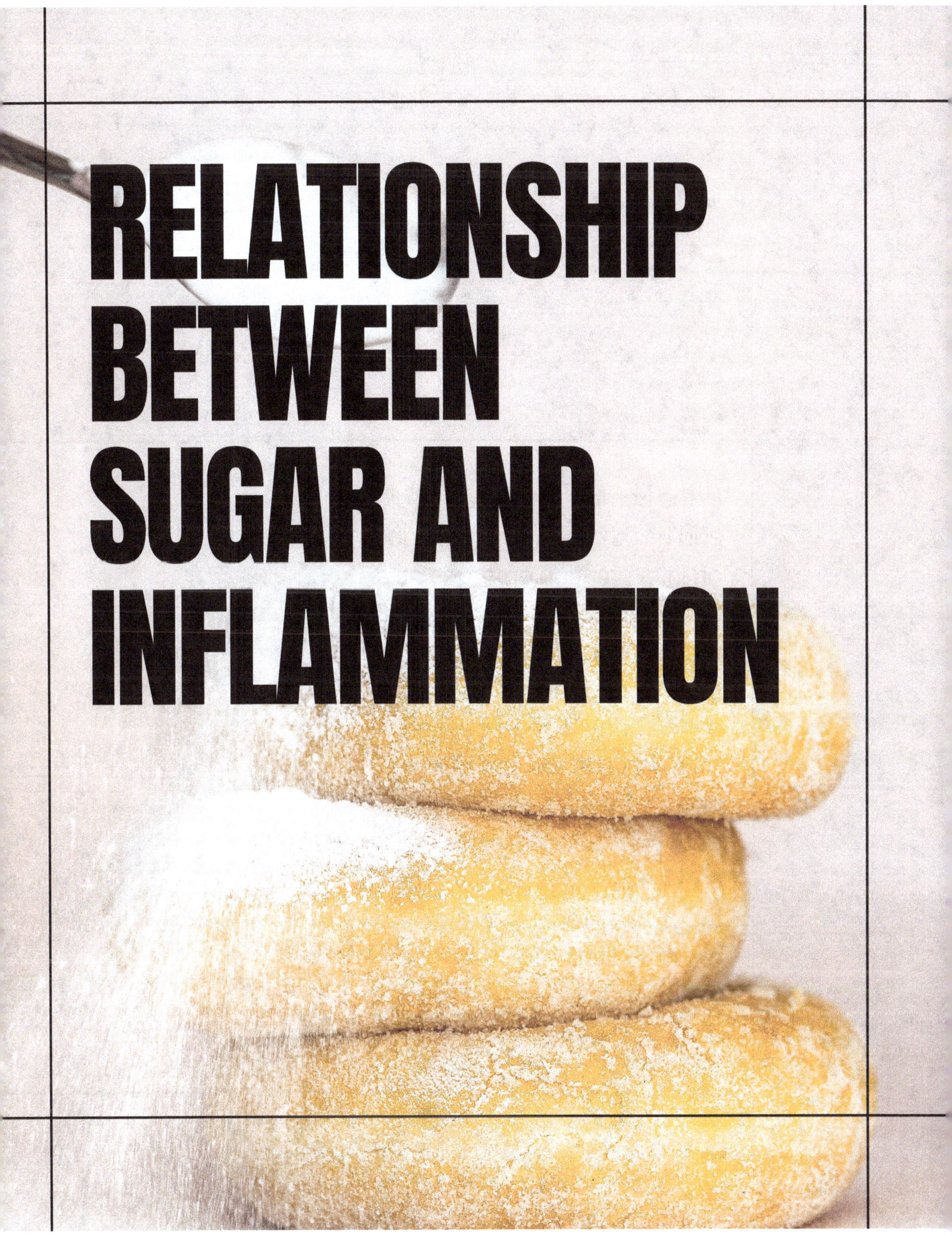

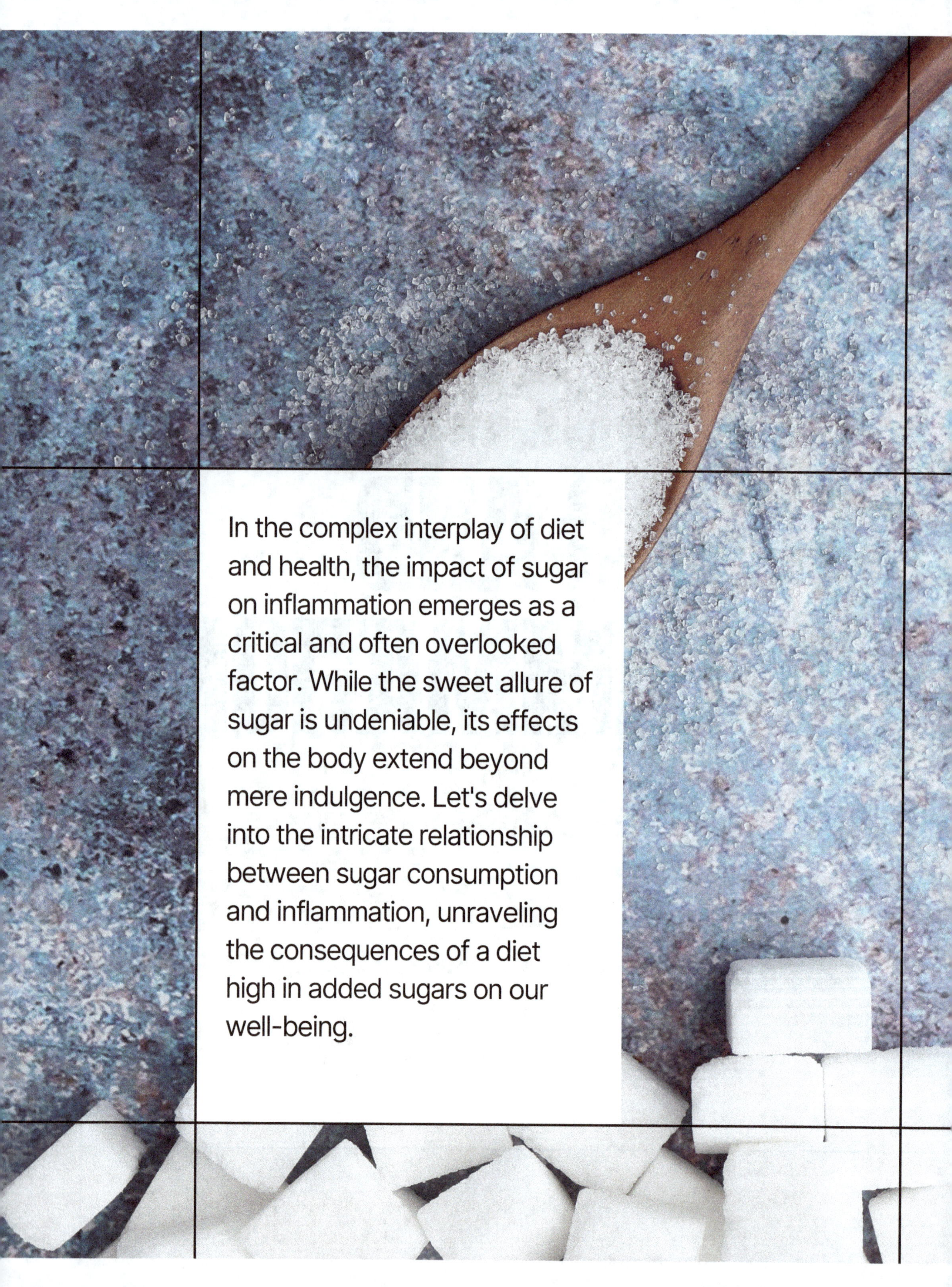

In the complex interplay of diet and health, the impact of sugar on inflammation emerges as a critical and often overlooked factor. While the sweet allure of sugar is undeniable, its effects on the body extend beyond mere indulgence. Let's delve into the intricate relationship between sugar consumption and inflammation, unraveling the consequences of a diet high in added sugars on our well-being.

The Sugar Landscape: Refined vs. Natural

To understand the inflammatory implications, it's important to differentiate between refined sugars and those naturally present in whole foods. Refined sugars, which are often found in processed foods and sugary beverages, are the main concern because they are quickly absorbed and can contribute to inflammation.

Blood Sugar Spikes: Inflammatory Triggers

Refined sugars cause rapid spikes in blood sugar levels, which triggers the release of insulin to regulate glucose. Chronically elevated insulin levels are linked to inflammation, which can become a recurring cycle, especially in diets dominated by sugary snacks and beverages.

Advanced Glycation End Products (AGEs):

Sugars attaching to proteins is called glycation. This process leads to the formation of Advanced Glycation End Products (AGEs). AGEs are abundant in diets high in added sugars and contribute to inflammation. They are also implicated in various age-related diseases.

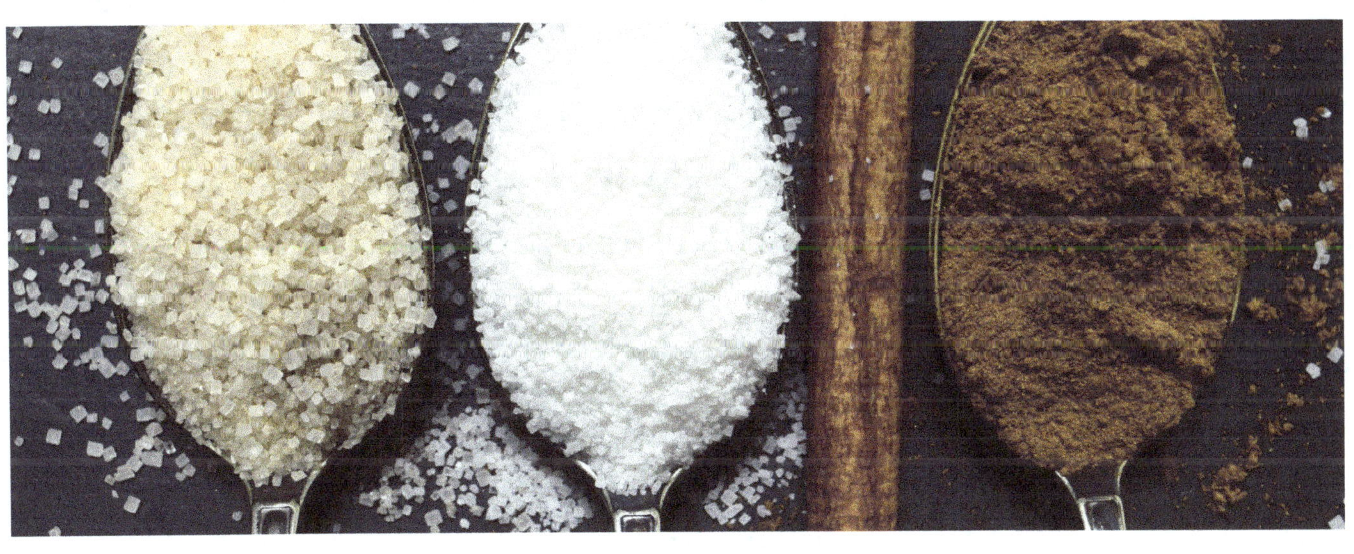

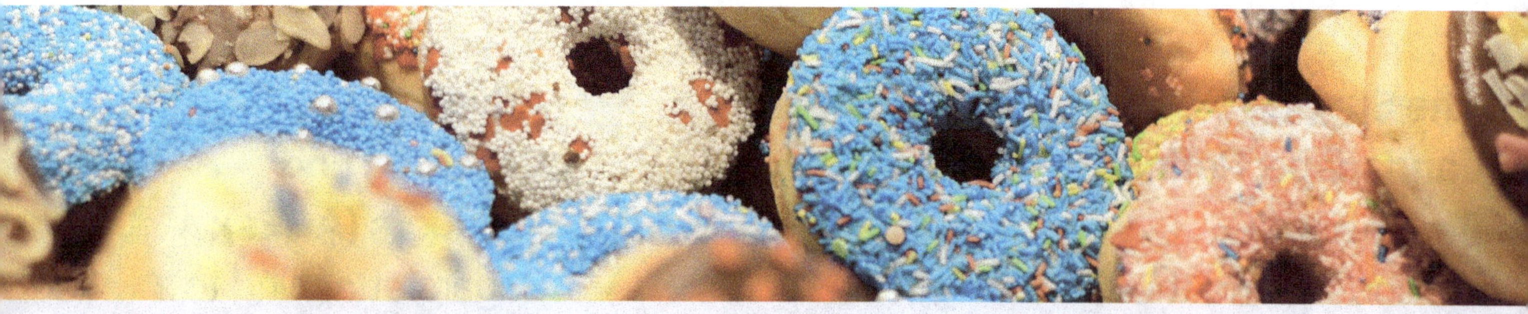

Pro-Inflammatory Cytokines: Sugar's Silent Instigators

A diet high in added sugars can increase the production of pro-inflammatory cytokines. These signaling molecules regulate inflammation, and elevated levels of them can contribute to a chronic inflammatory state. This sets the stage for various health issues.

Insulin Resistance

Persistent exposure to refined sugars can lead to insulin resistance. Insulin resistance is a precursor to conditions like type 2 diabetes and a driver of inflammation within the body.

Obesity: A Link to Systemic Inflammation

This connection between sugar and inflammation is intertwined with the rising rates of obesity. Excessive sugar intake contributes to weight gain. Adipose tissue secretes inflammatory substances, fostering a systemic inflammatory environment.

Joint Health: Sugar's Role in Inflammatory Conditions

Inflammation plays a significant role in joint-related conditions. Sugar consumption can negatively impact joint health by contributing to inflammatory processes that worsen conditions such as arthritis.

Cardiovascular Concerns: Sugar's Influence on Heart Health

The relationship between sugar and inflammation has significant implications for cardiovascular health. Diets high in added sugars may amplify the risk of heart disease by contributing to chronic inflammation.

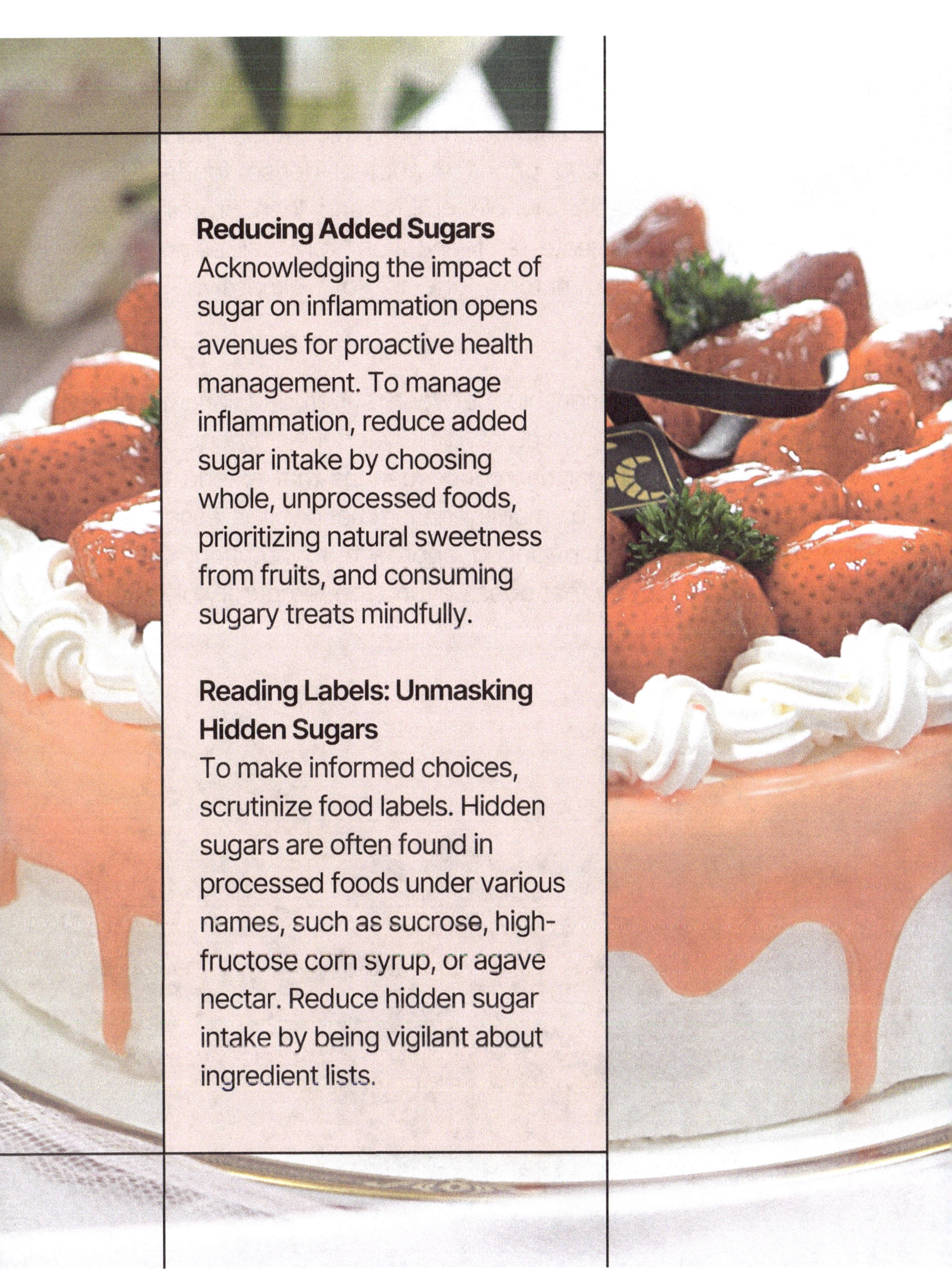

Reducing Added Sugars

Acknowledging the impact of sugar on inflammation opens avenues for proactive health management. To manage inflammation, reduce added sugar intake by choosing whole, unprocessed foods, prioritizing natural sweetness from fruits, and consuming sugary treats mindfully.

Reading Labels: Unmasking Hidden Sugars

To make informed choices, scrutinize food labels. Hidden sugars are often found in processed foods under various names, such as sucrose, high-fructose corn syrup, or agave nectar. Reduce hidden sugar intake by being vigilant about ingredient lists.

Balanced Eating: A Holistic Approach

To adopt a balanced and anti-inflammatory diet, it is important to reduce added sugars and prioritize nutrient-dense foods. This includes fruits, vegetables, whole grains, and lean proteins. By doing so, you can create a foundation for well-being that counteracts the inflammatory effects of excessive sugar consumption.

Understanding the relationship between sugar and inflammation reveals the significant impact of dietary choices on our health. Overconsumption of sugar has consequences that extend beyond momentary indulgence. To manage inflammation, it is essential to adopt a conscious and balanced approach to nutrition. Optimal health requires a journey that goes beyond the temporary pleasures of the sweet terrain.

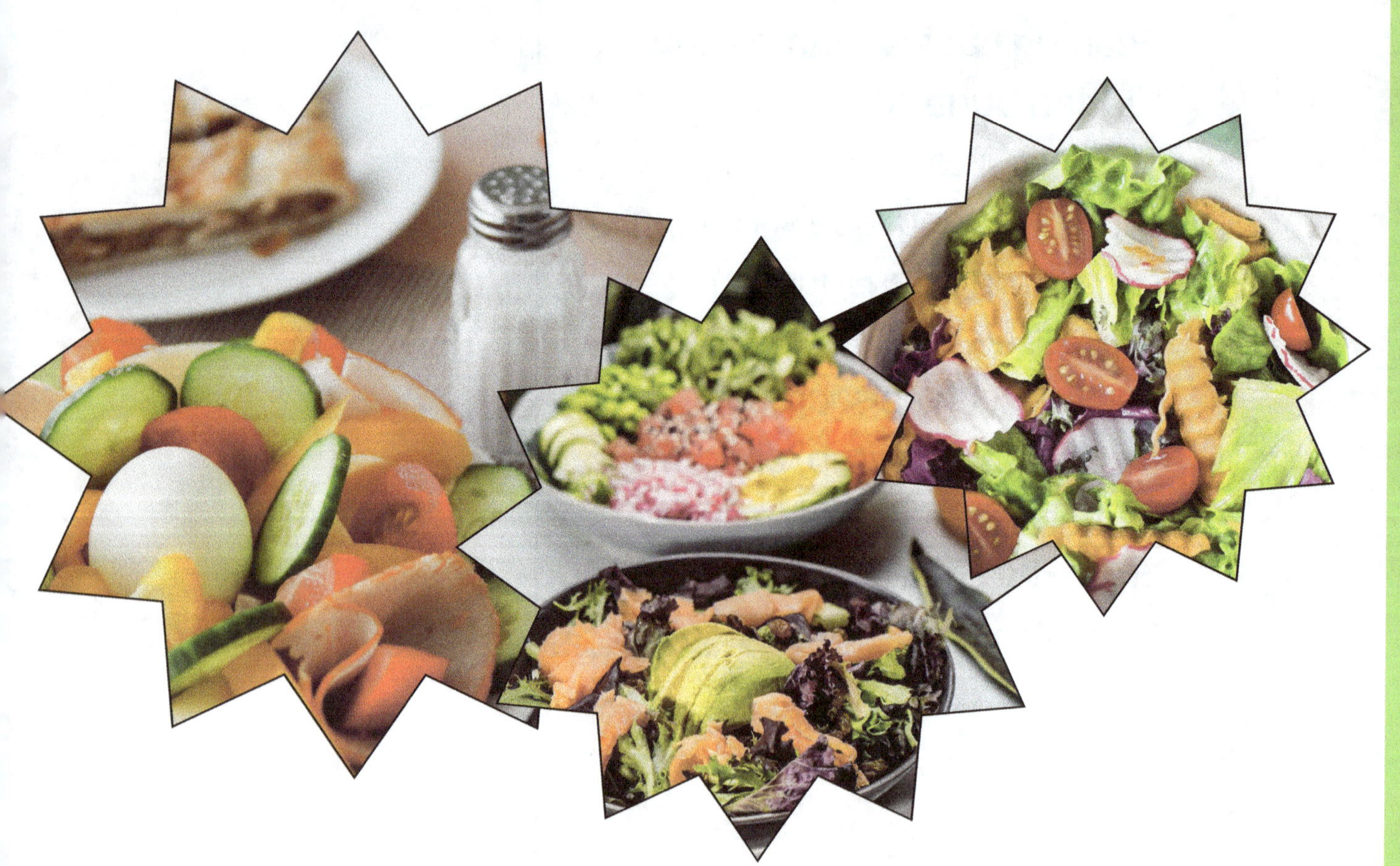

PROBIOTICS AND PREBIOTICS NOURISHING GUT HEALTH THROUGH DIET

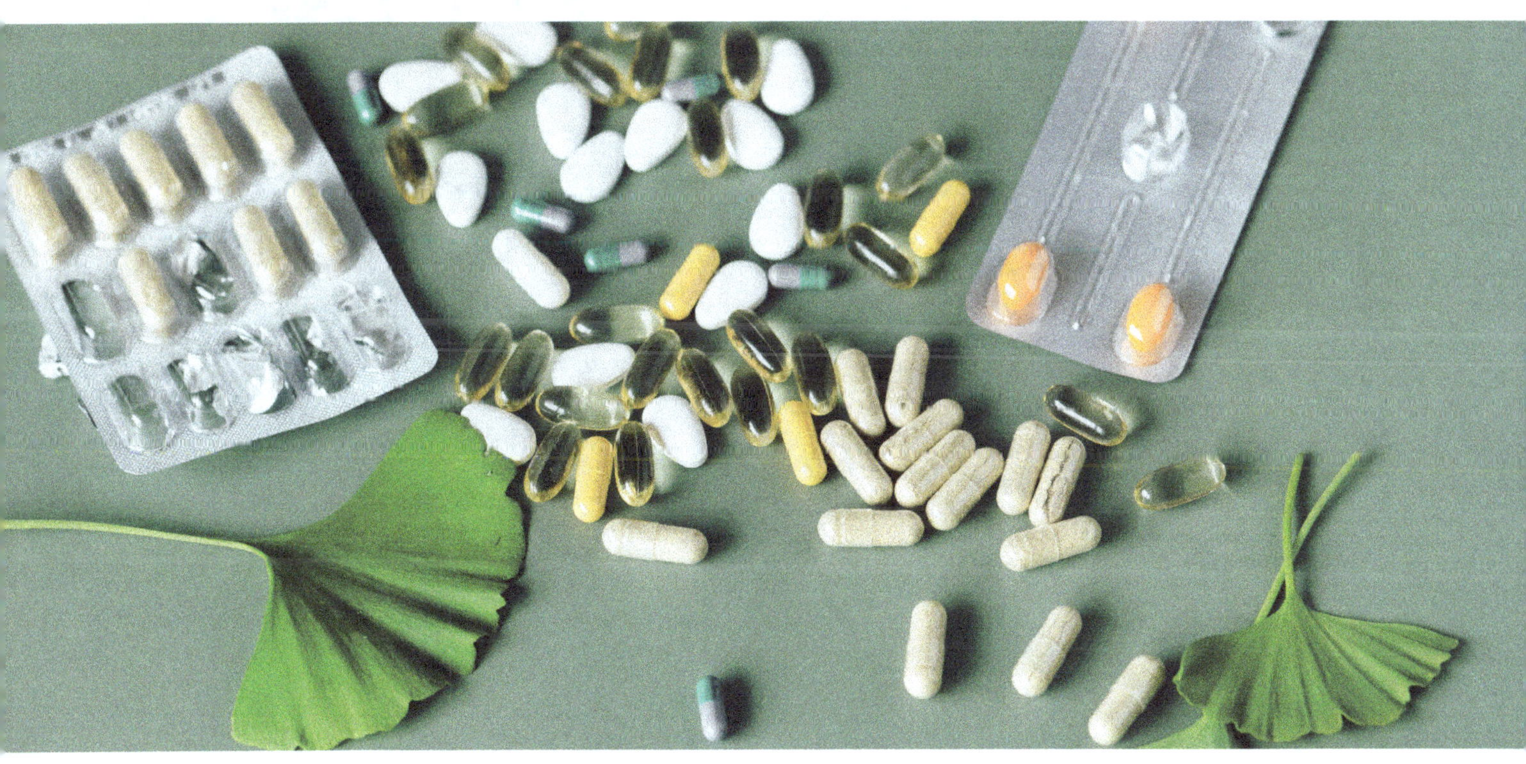

The ecosystem in our digestive tract is crucial for our well-being. Probiotics and prebiotics work together to support gut health and provide various health benefits. They contribute to digestive harmony and cultivate a resilient and thriving gut. Join us on a journey into the world of probiotics and prebiotics to learn more about how they work together.

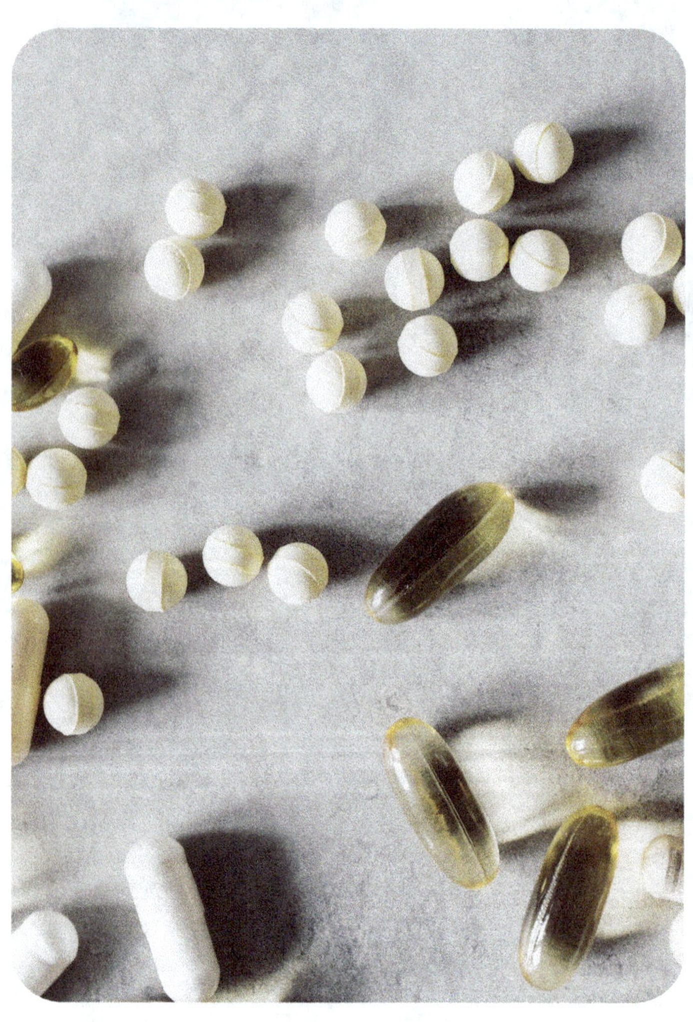

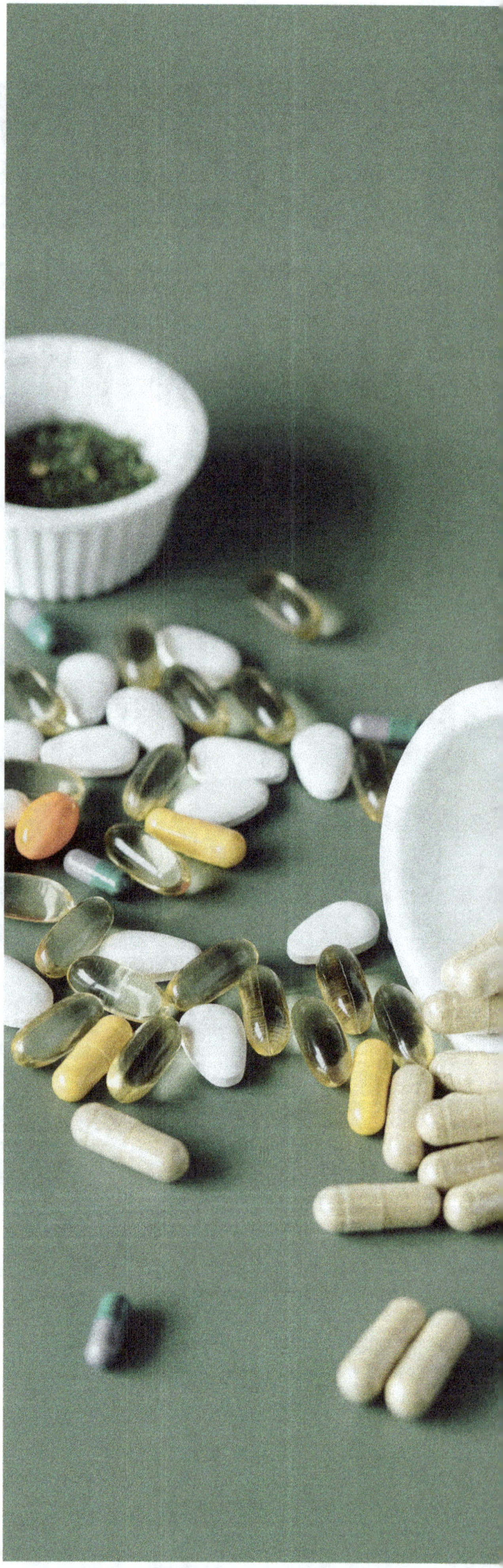

Probiotics: The Guardians of Gut Harmony

Probiotics are live microorganisms, such as bacteria and yeast, that provide health benefits when consumed in sufficient quantities. These friendly bacteria reside in the digestive tract, promoting a balanced microbial environment. Lactobacillus and Bifidobacterium are common probiotic strains, each with unique advantages for gut health.

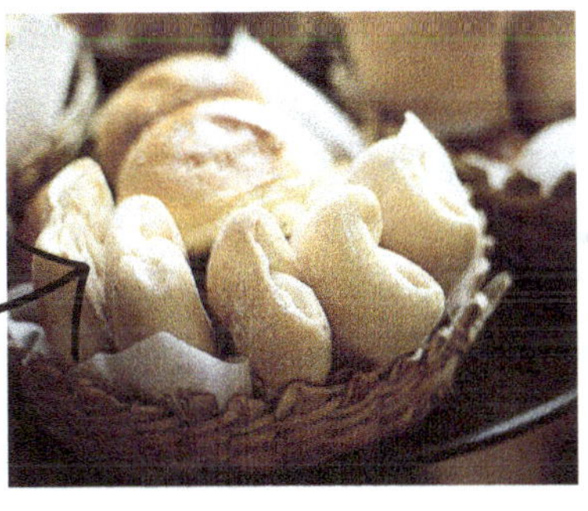

Fermented Foods: Nature's Probiotic Feast

Introducing probiotics into your diet is deliciously easy with fermented foods. Yogurt, kefir, sauerkraut, kimchi, and miso are all culinary delights that are teeming with live cultures. By incorporating these foods into your meals, you can add depth to flavors and infuse your gut with beneficial probiotics.

Supplements: Precision in Probiotic Intake

Supplements are a convenient option for those seeking a more targeted approach to probiotic consumption. Probiotic capsules or powders provide specific strains in controlled doses, allowing for personalized gut health support. It is recommended to consult with a healthcare professional to determine the most suitable probiotic supplement for individual needs.

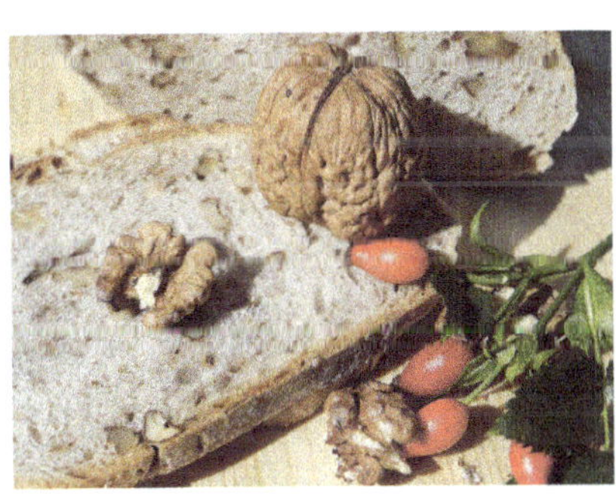

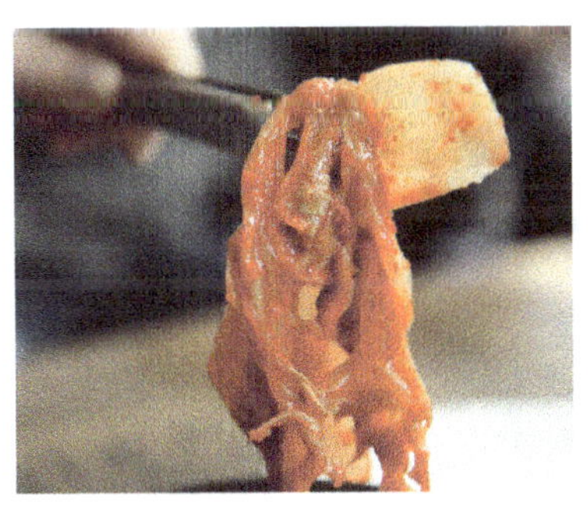

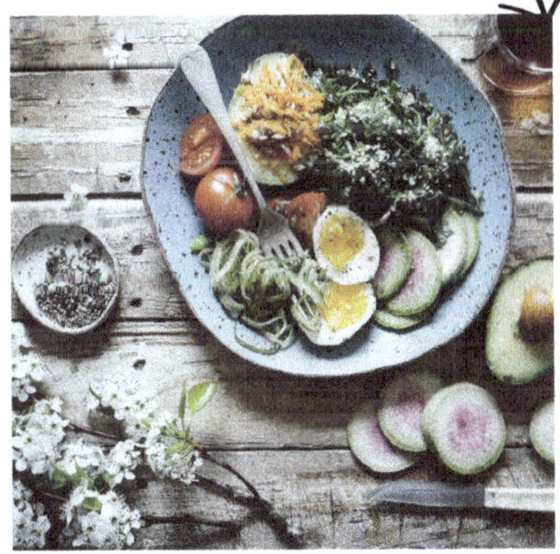

Diverse Strains for Comprehensive Support

The diversity of probiotic strains reflects the complexity of the gut microbiome. Including a variety of probiotic-rich foods or supplements introduces different strains, enhancing overall gut microbial diversity. This diversity is associated with improved digestion and a stronger immune system.

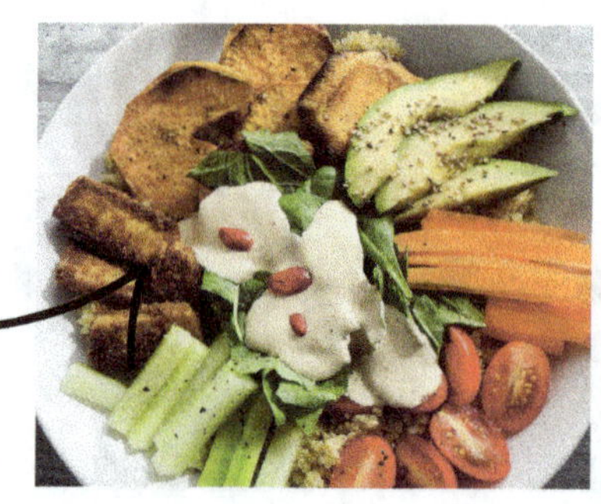

Prebiotics: The Fuel for Gut Microbes

Prebiotics are fibers that cannot be digested and serve as food for beneficial bacteria in the gut. They are found in fruits, vegetables, and whole grains and stimulate the growth and activity of probiotics. This relationship between prebiotics and probiotics creates a harmonious environment in the gut.

Fiber-Rich Foods: Nurturing Gut Microbes Naturally

Fiber-rich whole foods like bananas, onions, garlic, leeks, asparagus, and oats are excellent sources of prebiotics. Probiotics feast on these undigested fibers in the colon, making them an essential part of a healthy gut. Including a variety of fiber-rich foods in your diet can naturally boost gut health.

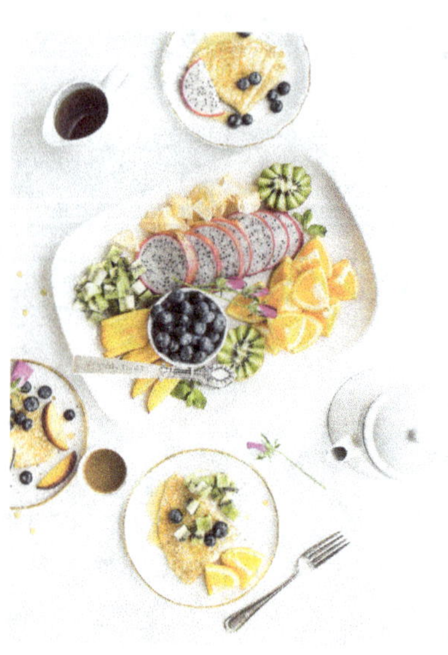

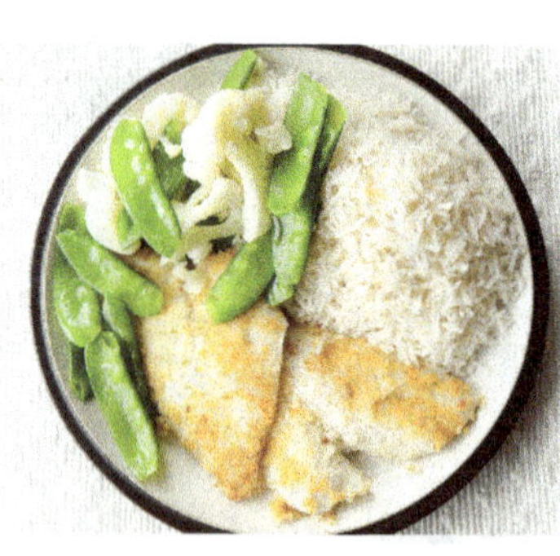

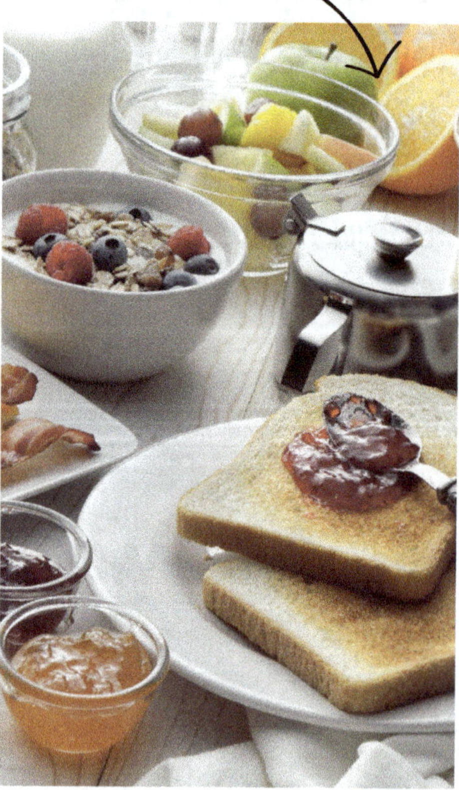

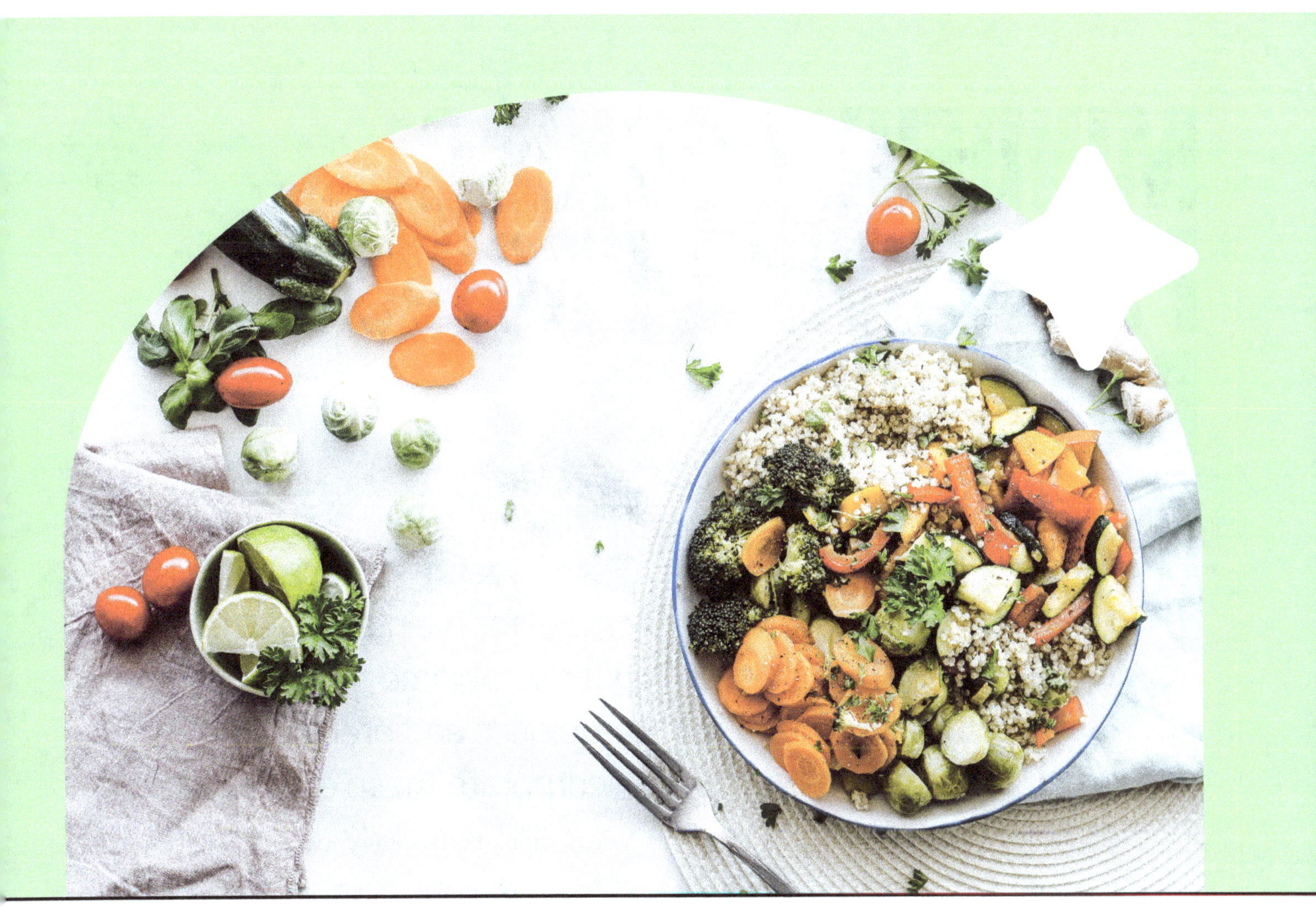

Balancing Act: Probiotics, Prebiotics, and Your Plate - To achieve a balanced and gut-friendly diet, make intentional choices. You can create a symbiotic relationship by pairing probiotic-rich foods with prebiotic sources, which fosters the growth and activity of beneficial microbes. For instance, you can enjoy yogurt with a sprinkle of oats or add sautéed garlic and onions to your favorite dishes.

Gut-Healing Herbs: Nature's Prebiotics - Certain herbs, such as dandelion greens, chicory root, and garlic, contain compounds that act as prebiotics. These natural additions can infuse dishes with flavor and provide gut-friendly support. It is important to note that these herbs should be used in moderation to avoid any adverse effects.

MINDFUL COOKING: PRESERVING PROBIOTIC POTENCY

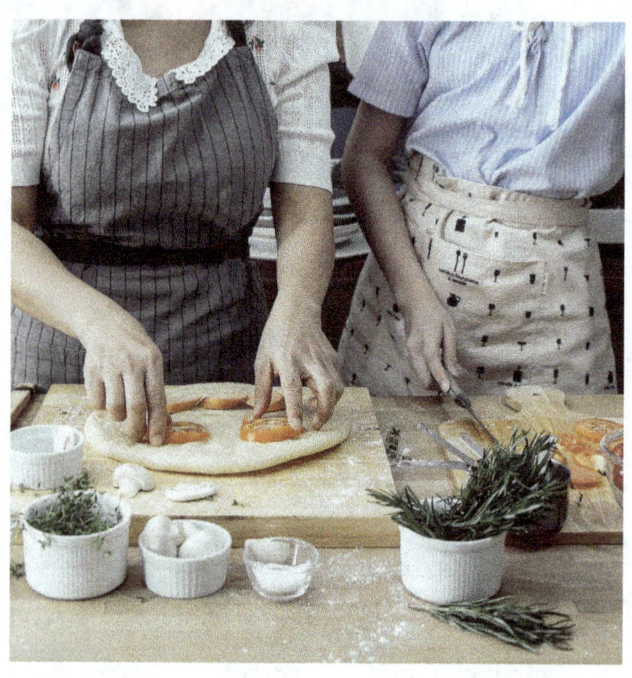

Maintaining Balance for Long-Term Health - Consistency is crucial for maintaining a healthy gut microbiome through the use of probiotics and prebiotics. Incorporate these elements into your diet regularly to promote digestive well-being, overall health, and immune resilience over time.

Cooking can change probiotics' structure, but some heat-resistant strains can withstand mild cooking. To maximize benefits, add probiotic-rich foods to recipes that don't involve high heat. For example, add fermented toppings to salads or incorporate probiotic-rich yogurt into dips.

Probiotics and prebiotics promote gut health and improve overall well-being. They influence digestion and various health factors. A diet rich in probiotic and prebiotic foods creates an environment where beneficial microorganisms thrive, leading to a stronger immune system and better digestion.

HOW PHYTONUTRIENTS FIGHT INFLAMMATION

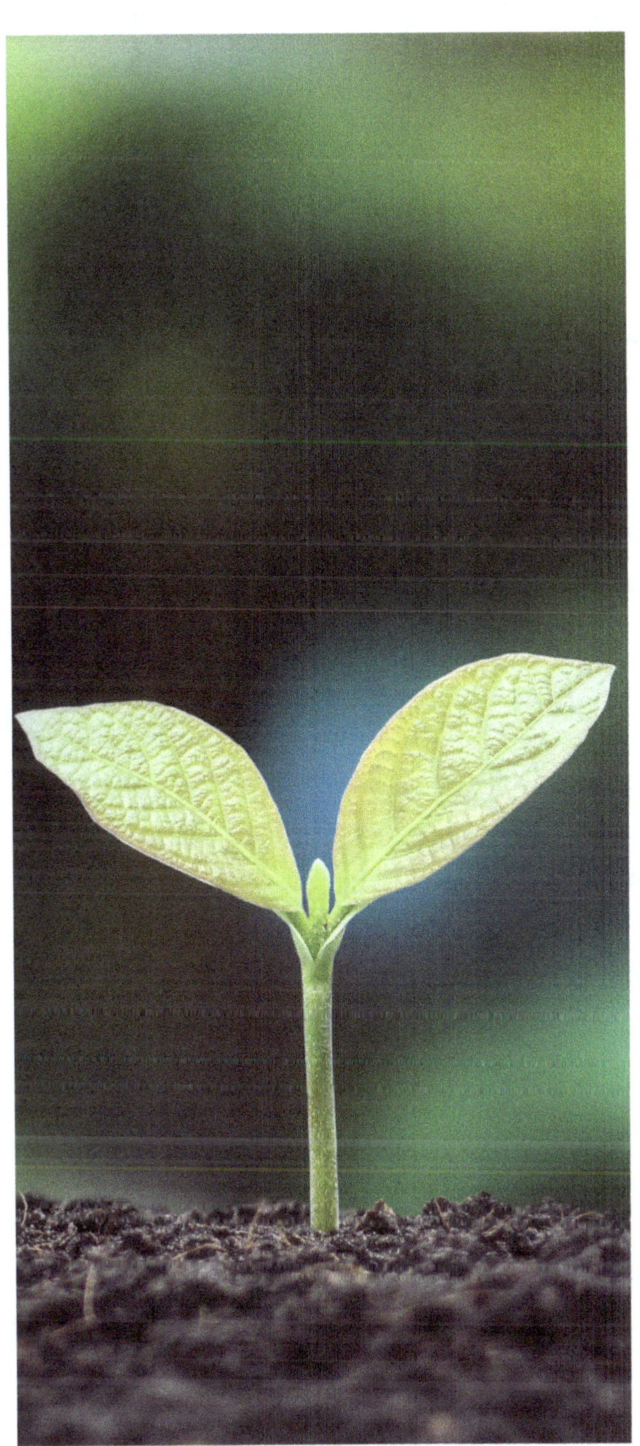

Phytonutrients are bioactive compounds derived from plants that can combat inflammation in the body. In the realm of nutrition, they are important defenders that go beyond simple nourishment. They offer a variety of colors, flavors, and health benefits. This text explores the fascinating world of phytonutrients and how they contribute to fighting inflammation.

Diverse Array of Phytonutrients - Plant-based foods contain a variety of phytonutrients, such as flavonoids, carotenoids, glucosinolates, and polyphenols. These compounds have unique properties that collectively contribute to the anti-inflammatory effects of these foods.

Flavonoids: Nature's Anti-Inflammatory Agents - Flavonoids are celebrated for their antioxidant and anti-inflammatory properties. They are abundant in fruits, vegetables, tea, and dark chocolate. Examples of flavonoids that actively combat inflammation at the cellular level include quercetin in apples, catechins in green tea, and anthocyanins in berries.

Carotenoids: Colorful Guardians of Health - The vibrant hues of orange, red, and green in fruits and vegetables signify the presence of carotenoids. Beta-carotene in carrots, lycopene in tomatoes, and lutein in leafy greens contribute not only to the visual appeal of foods but also to their anti-inflammatory and antioxidant effects.

Polyphenols: Versatile Defenders - Polyphenols are versatile compounds found in many plant foods. They have anti-inflammatory properties. Grapes contain resveratrol, turmeric contains curcumin, and green tea contains epigallocatechin gallate (EGCG). These diverse polyphenols play a crucial role in modulating inflammatory responses.

Glucosinolates: Cruciferous Champions - Broccoli, kale, and Brussels sprouts are cruciferous vegetables that are rich in glucosinolates. These compounds break down during digestion and produce sulforaphane, which is known for its anti-inflammatory and potential cancer-fighting properties.

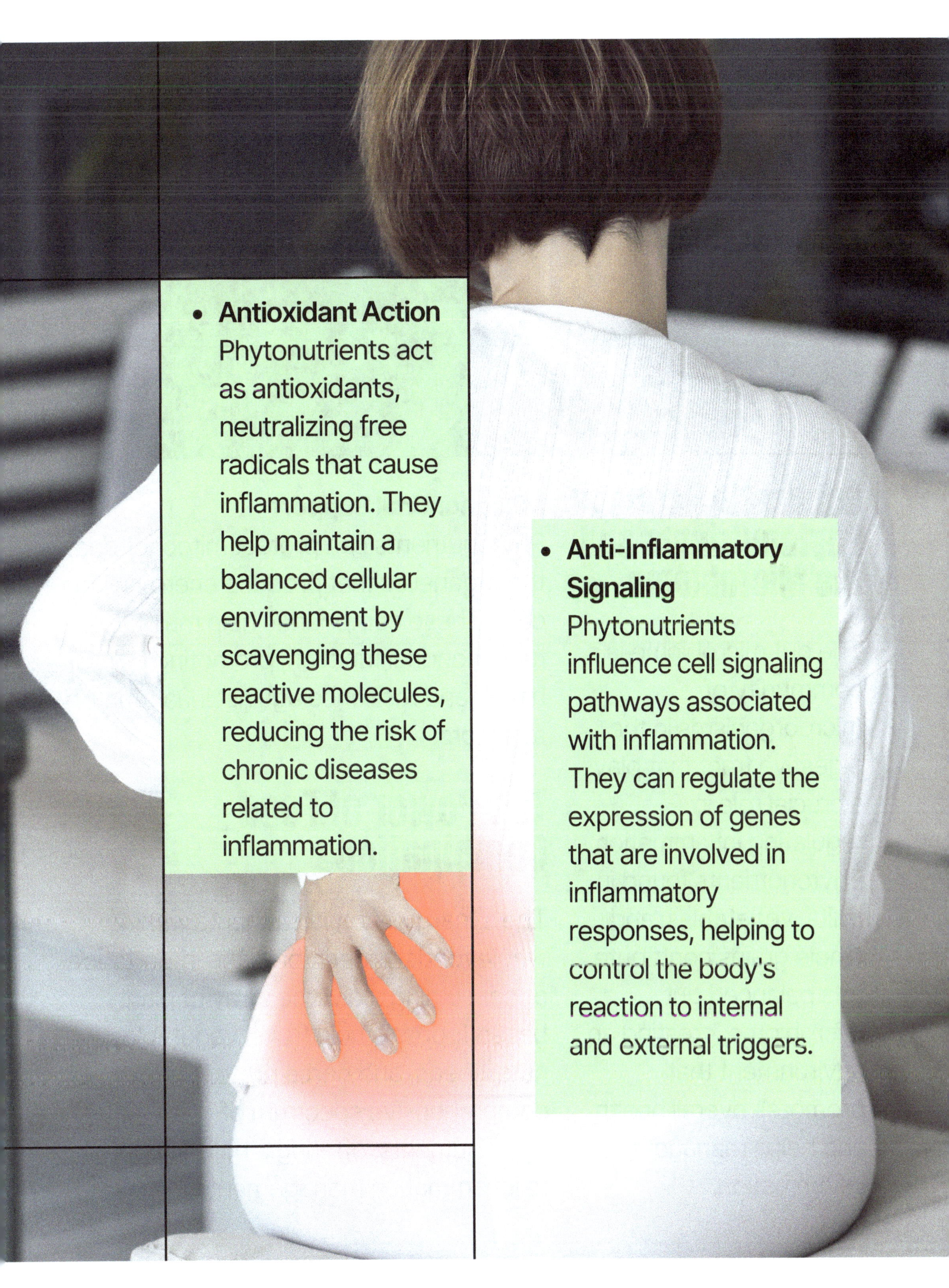

Antioxidant Action Phytonutrients act as antioxidants, neutralizing free radicals that cause inflammation. They help maintain a balanced cellular environment by scavenging these reactive molecules, reducing the risk of chronic diseases related to inflammation.

Anti-Inflammatory Signaling Phytonutrients influence cell signaling pathways associated with inflammation. They can regulate the expression of genes that are involved in inflammatory responses, helping to control the body's reaction to internal and external triggers.

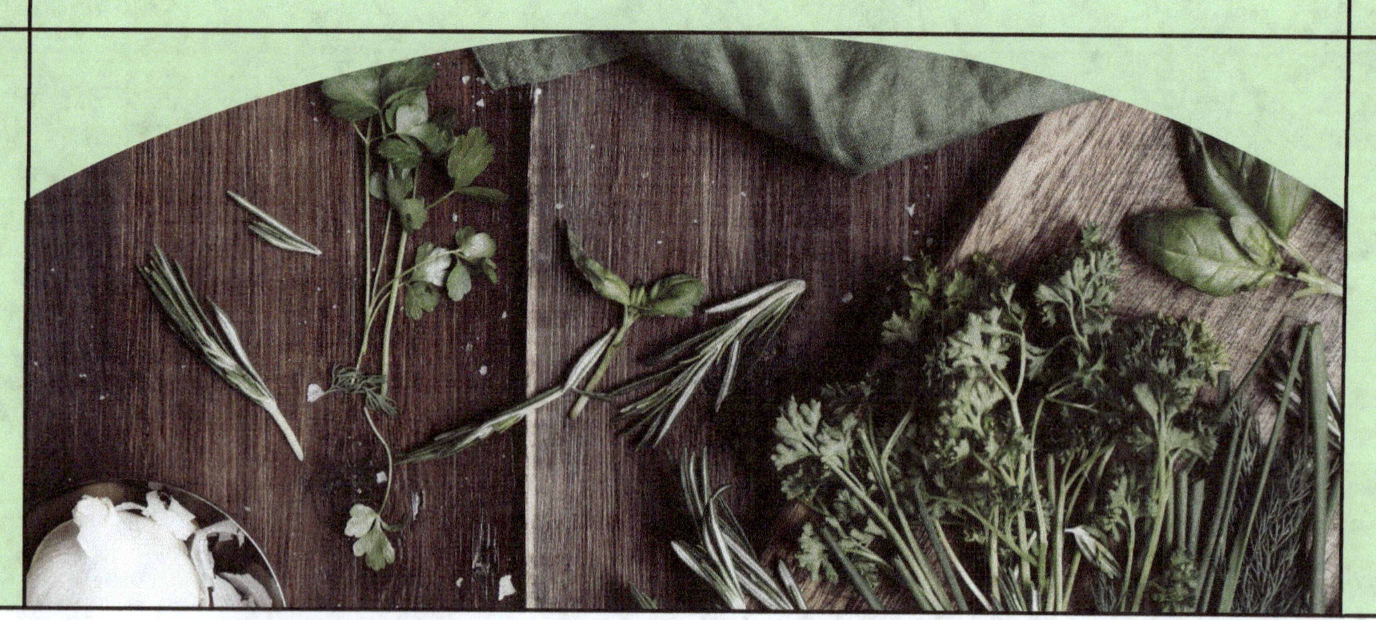

Gut Health Harmony: Phytonutrients and the Microbiome

The gut microbiome is a community of microorganisms in the digestive tract that plays a crucial role in regulating inflammation. Phytonutrients found in fruits, vegetables, and whole grains contribute to a balanced gut microbiome, creating an environment that promotes overall health and helps manage inflammation.

Mitochondrial Support

Phytonutrients can protect mitochondria, the organelles that produce energy within cells. These compounds help maintain mitochondrial function, promoting cellular health and resilience against inflammatory stressors.

The Power of Food Combinations

The synergy of phytonutrients within whole foods underscores the importance of consuming a diverse array of plant-based foods. Whole fruits, vegetables, nuts, seeds, and herbs provide a comprehensive spectrum of phytonutrients, offering a holistic approach to inflammation management.

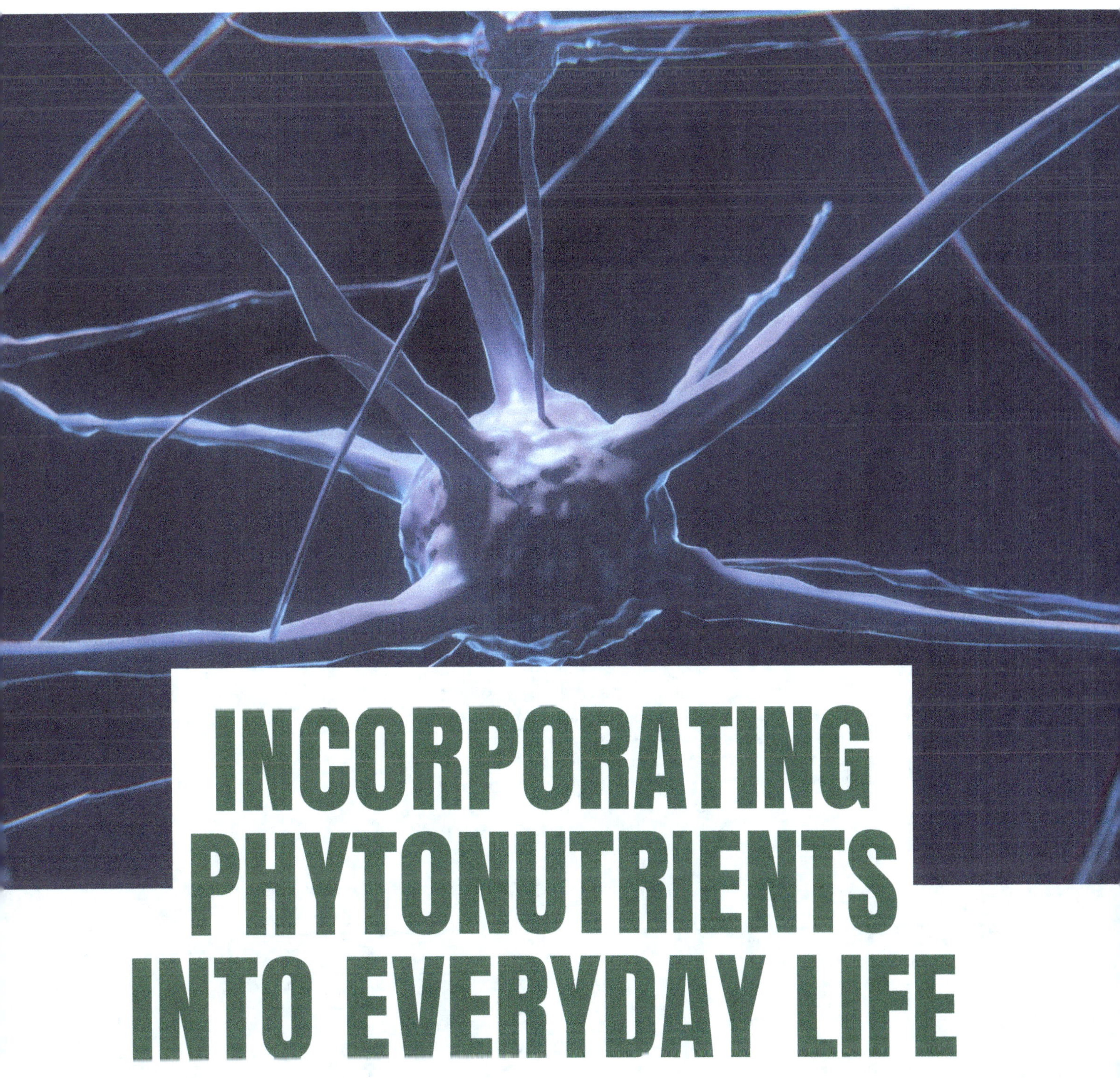

INCORPORATING PHYTONUTRIENTS INTO EVERYDAY LIFE

Mitochondrial Support Phytonutrients can protect mitochondria, the organelles that produce energy within cells. These compounds help maintain mitochondrial function, promoting cellular health and resilience against inflammatory stressors.

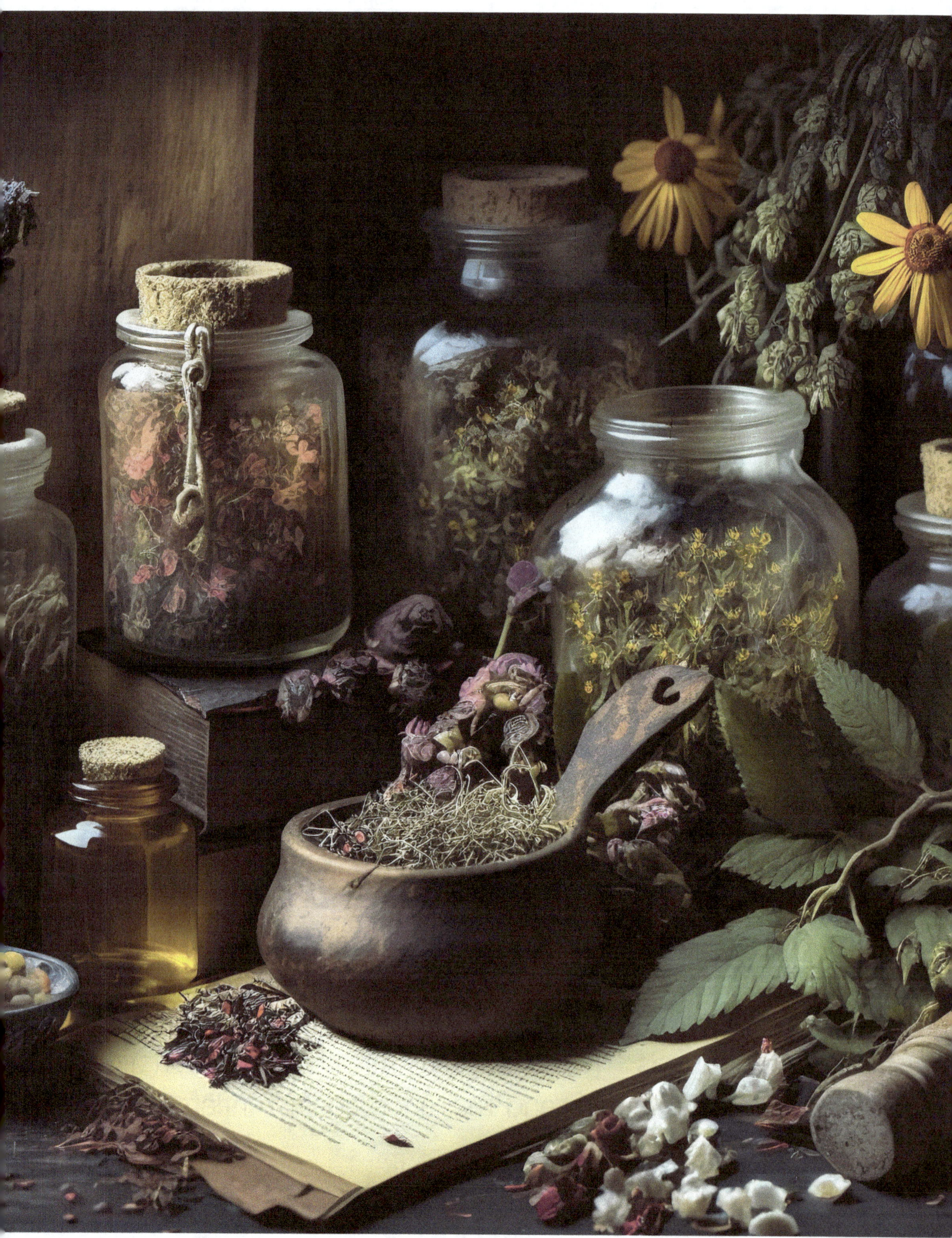

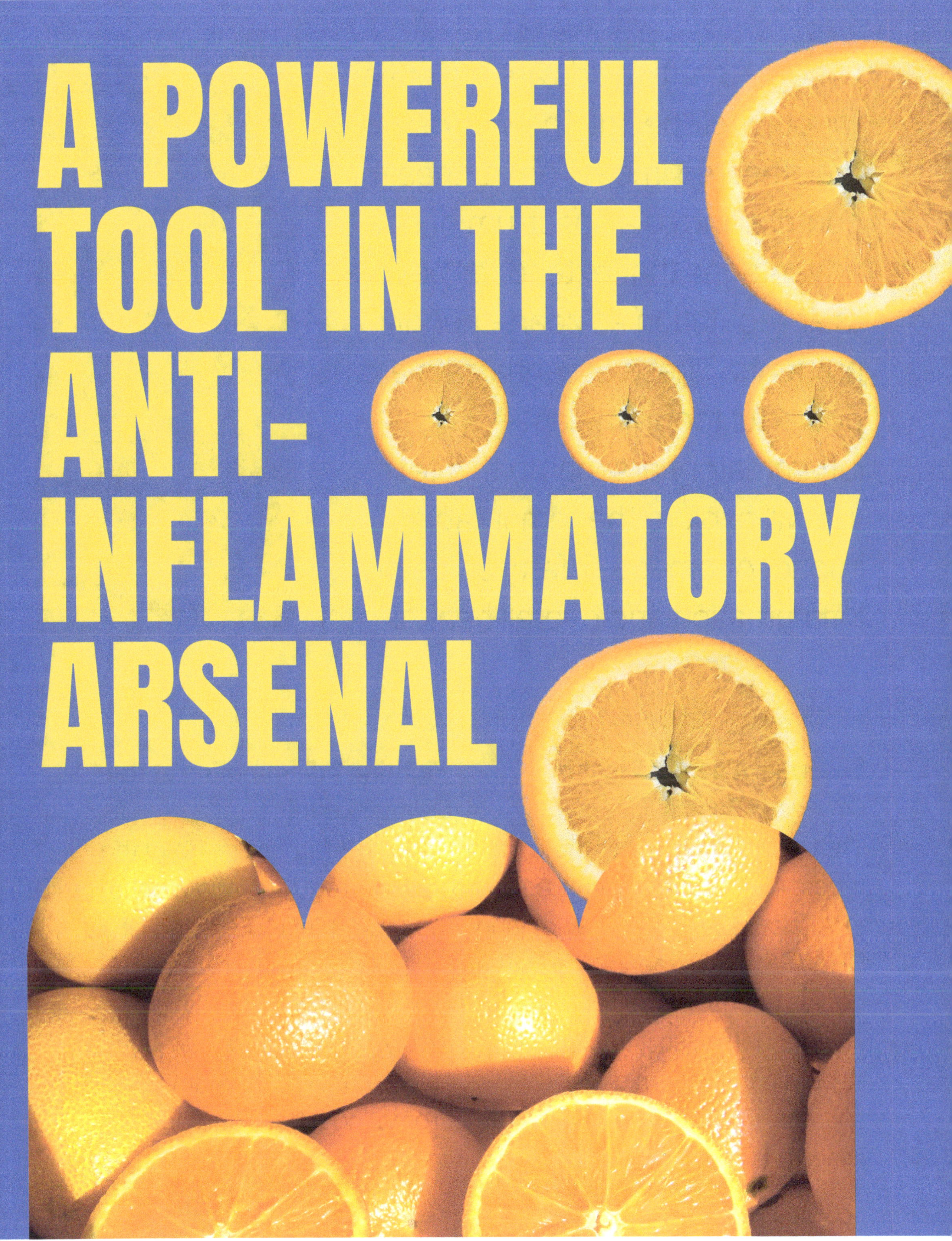
A POWERFUL TOOL IN THE ANTI-INFLAMMATORY ARSENAL

Omega-3 fatty acids are essential for our well-being. They have a multifaceted impact on our health, contributing to a spectrum of health advantages that extend far beyond their reputation as heart-friendly nutrients. These essential fats are a powerful tool in the anti-inflammatory arsenal. In this text, we will explore the remarkable impact of omega-3 fatty acids on inflammation and overall health.

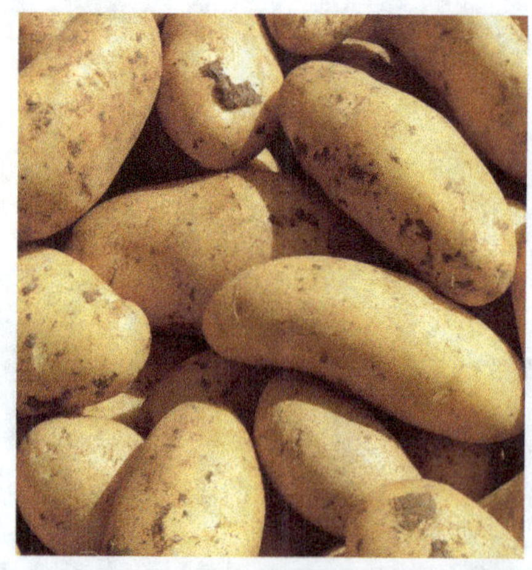

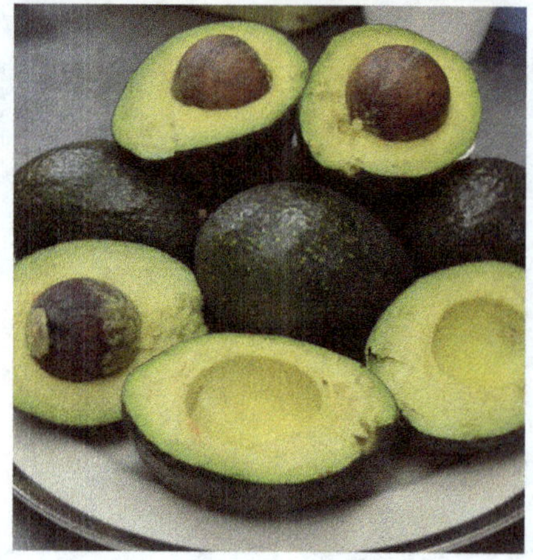

Essential Allies for Health: Omega-3 Basics

They are classified into three main types: ALA (alpha-linolenic acid), EPA (eicosapentaenoic acid), and DHA (docosahexaenoic acid). Our bodies cannot produce them independently, so it is important to obtain them from dietary sources. Omega-3 fatty acids are essential for optimal health.

Fighting Inflammation at the Cellular Level

Omega-3 fatty acids have the ability to regulate inflammation at the cellular level. EPA and DHA are particularly important in producing specialized pro-resolving mediators (SPMs) that actively resolve inflammation, promoting a balanced and controlled response.

Brain Boost: Omega-3s and Cognitive Function

Omega-3s, particularly DHA, benefit the brain, which is rich in fats. These fatty acids are essential to the structure of cell membranes and support neurotransmitter function. Studies suggest that omega-3s may help maintain cognitive health and reduce the risk of age-related cognitive decline.

Mood Modulators: Omega-3s and Mental Well-Being

Emerging research suggests that omega-3 fatty acids may have a positive impact on mental health, potentially benefiting those with conditions such as depression and anxiety. These fats have anti-inflammatory and neuroprotective properties that can promote emotional well-being and a positive mood.

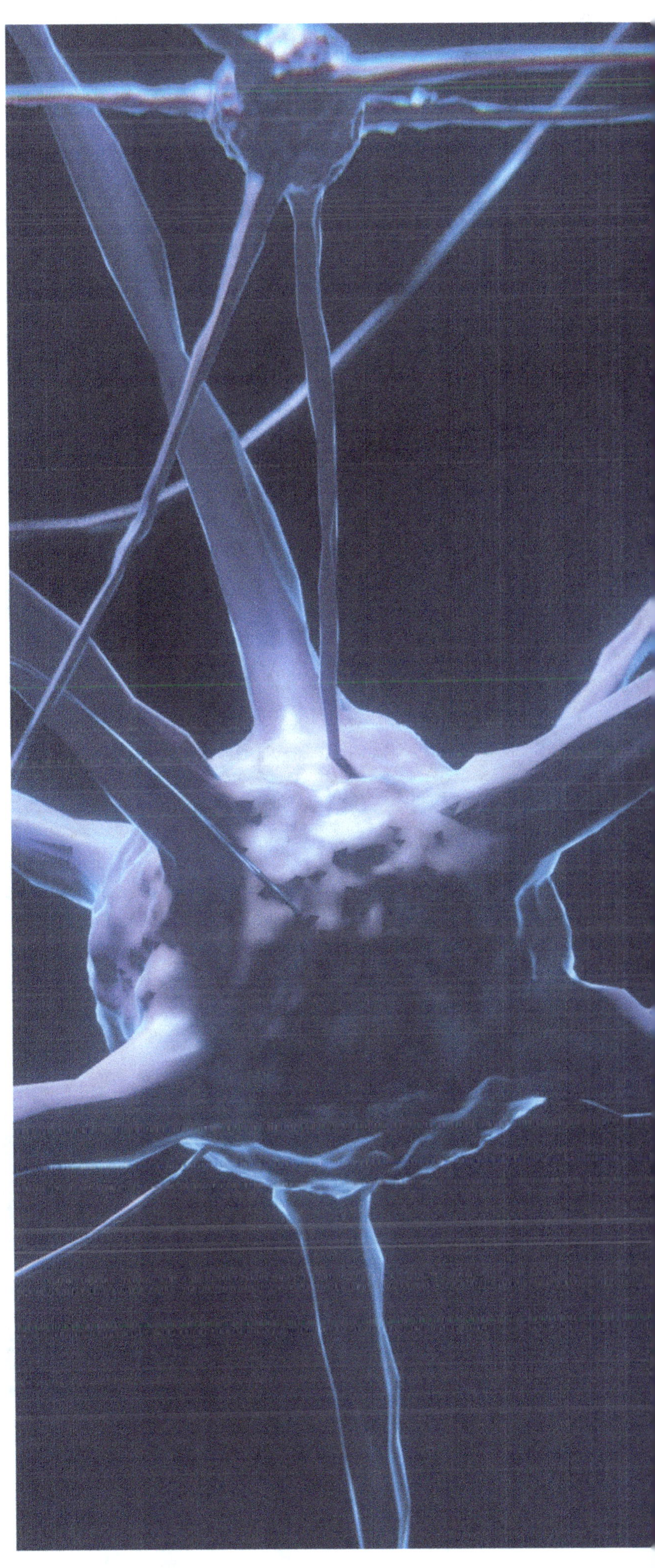

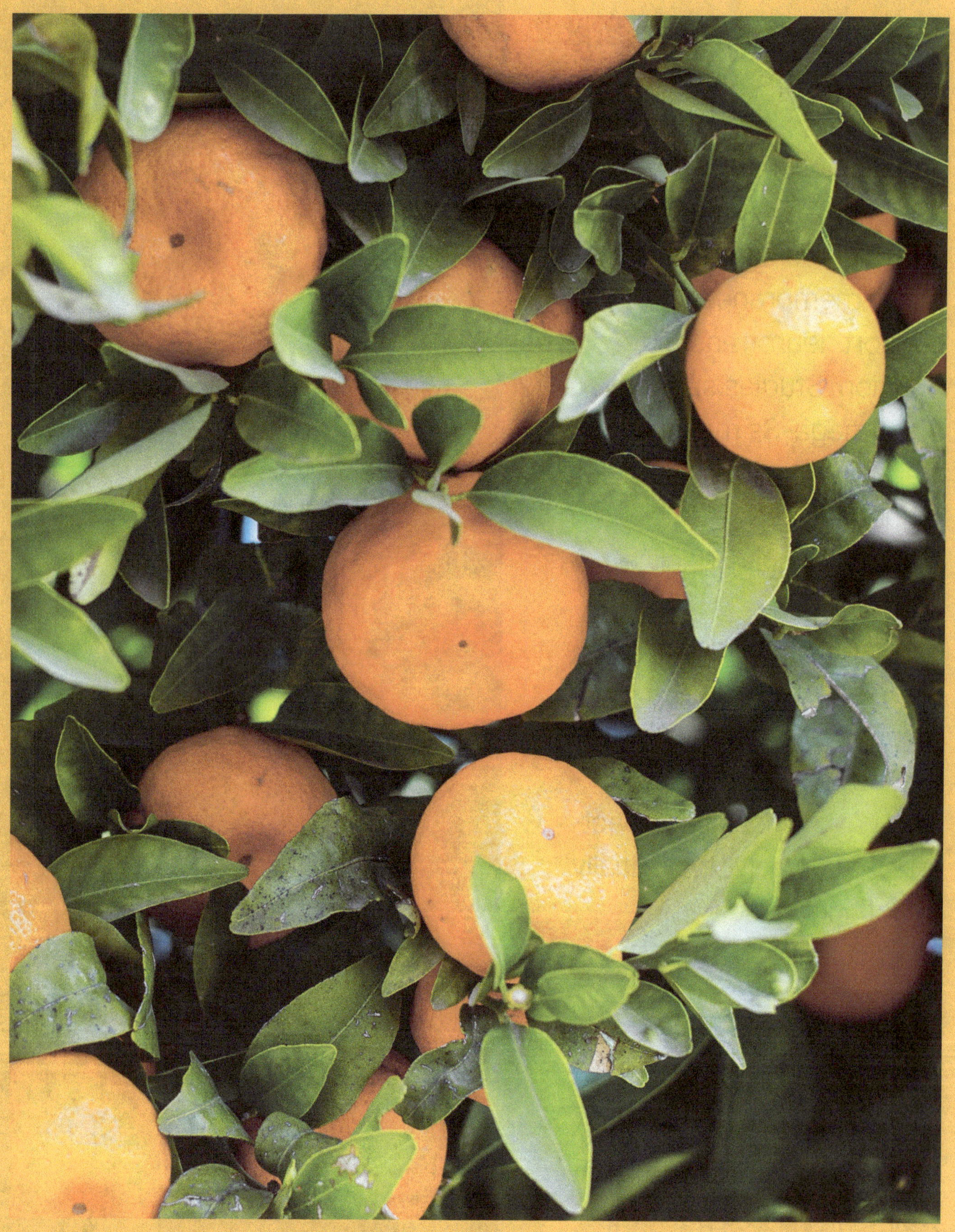

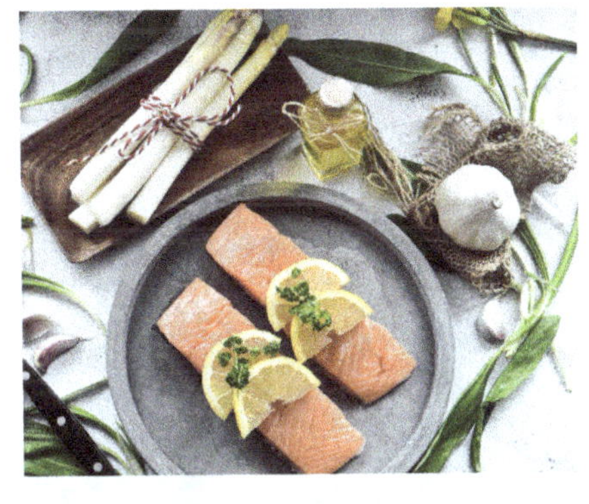

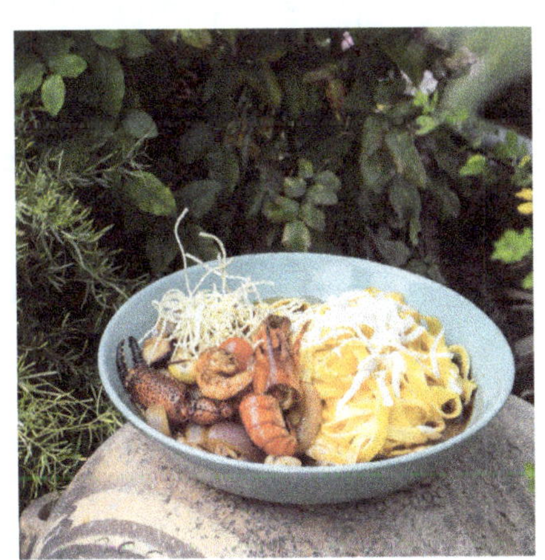

Maintaining a balanced ratio of omega-3 to omega-6 fatty acids is essential for optimal health. The Western diet, often high in omega-6 fatty acids from vegetable oils, can disrupt this balance. Increasing omega-3 intake helps restore equilibrium, promoting an anti-inflammatory state within the body.

Supplements: Bridging the Nutritional Gap

For those seeking to augment their omega-3 intake, supplements such as fish oil capsules or algae based supplements offer a convenient solution. Consultation with a healthcare professional can guide the appropriate dosage based on individual health needs.

Omega-3s with Environmental Awareness

As we embrace the benefits of omega-3 fatty acids, it's crucial to make sustainable choices. Opting for sustainably sourced fish and eco-friendly omega-3 supplements aligns our health goals with a commitment to environmental well-being.

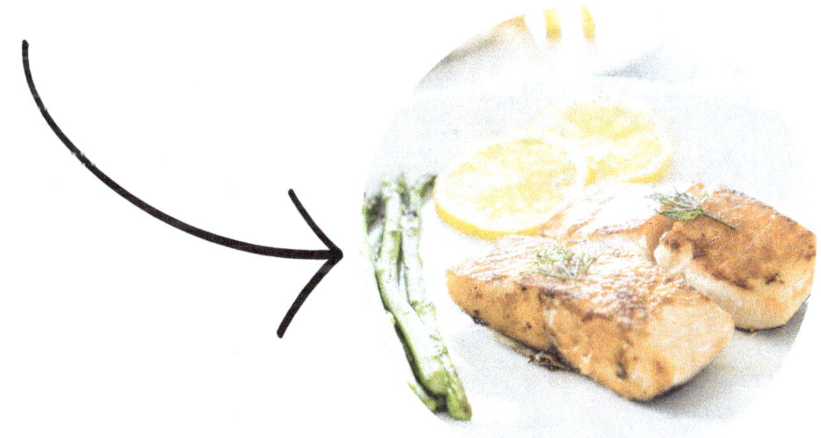

A TRENDY APPROACH TO INFLAMMATION REDUCTION

INTERMITTENT FASTING

Intermittent fasting, a dietary pattern that alternates between periods of eating and fasting, has gained attention not only for its potential to manage weight, but also for its intriguing effects on inflammation in the body.

Beyond the traditional realm of dietary approaches, intermittent fasting is emerging as a powerful strategy for recalibrating the body's inflammatory responses and promoting overall health.

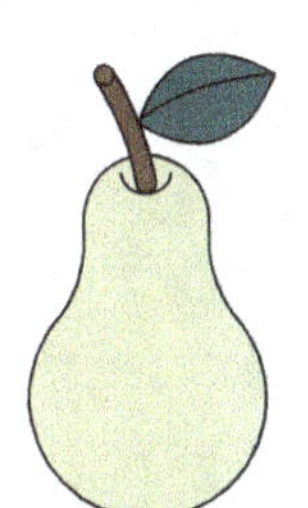

Understanding Intermittent Fasting - A Paradigm Shift in Eating Patterns:

Intermittent fasting is not about specific food choices, but rather about when to eat. It encompasses several methods, including the 16/8 method (16 hours of fasting with an 8-hour eating window), the 5:2 method (alternating between regular eating and two days of reduced caloric intake), and the eat-stop-eat method (24-hour fasting periods once or twice a week).

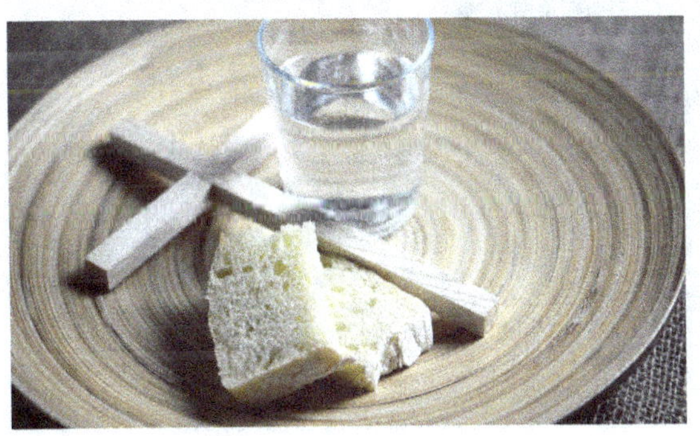

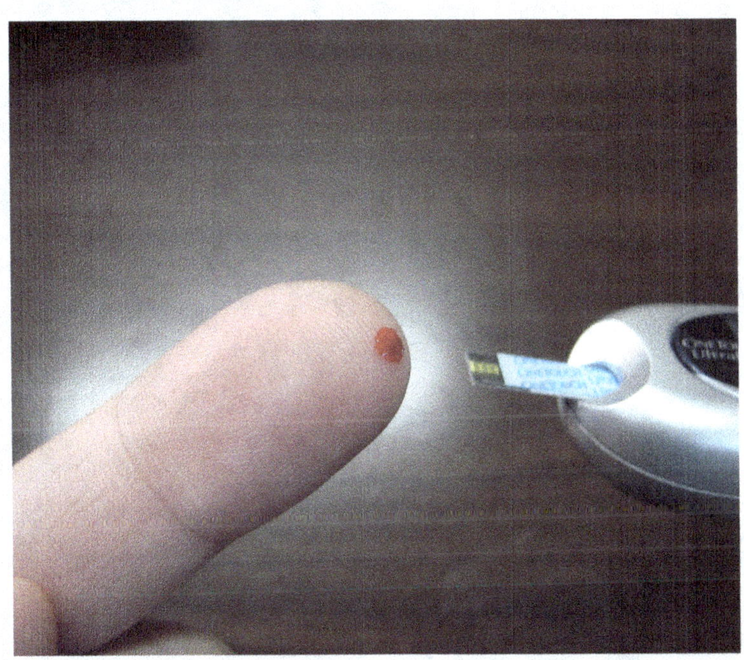

Metabolic Reset: Balancing Blood Sugar Levels:

One of the key anti-inflammatory mechanisms of intermittent fasting is its ability to regulate blood glucose levels. Fasting periods prompt the body to use stored glucose, reducing the frequency of blood sugar spikes and creating a more stable metabolic environment. This stability contributes to a reduced inflammatory response in the body.

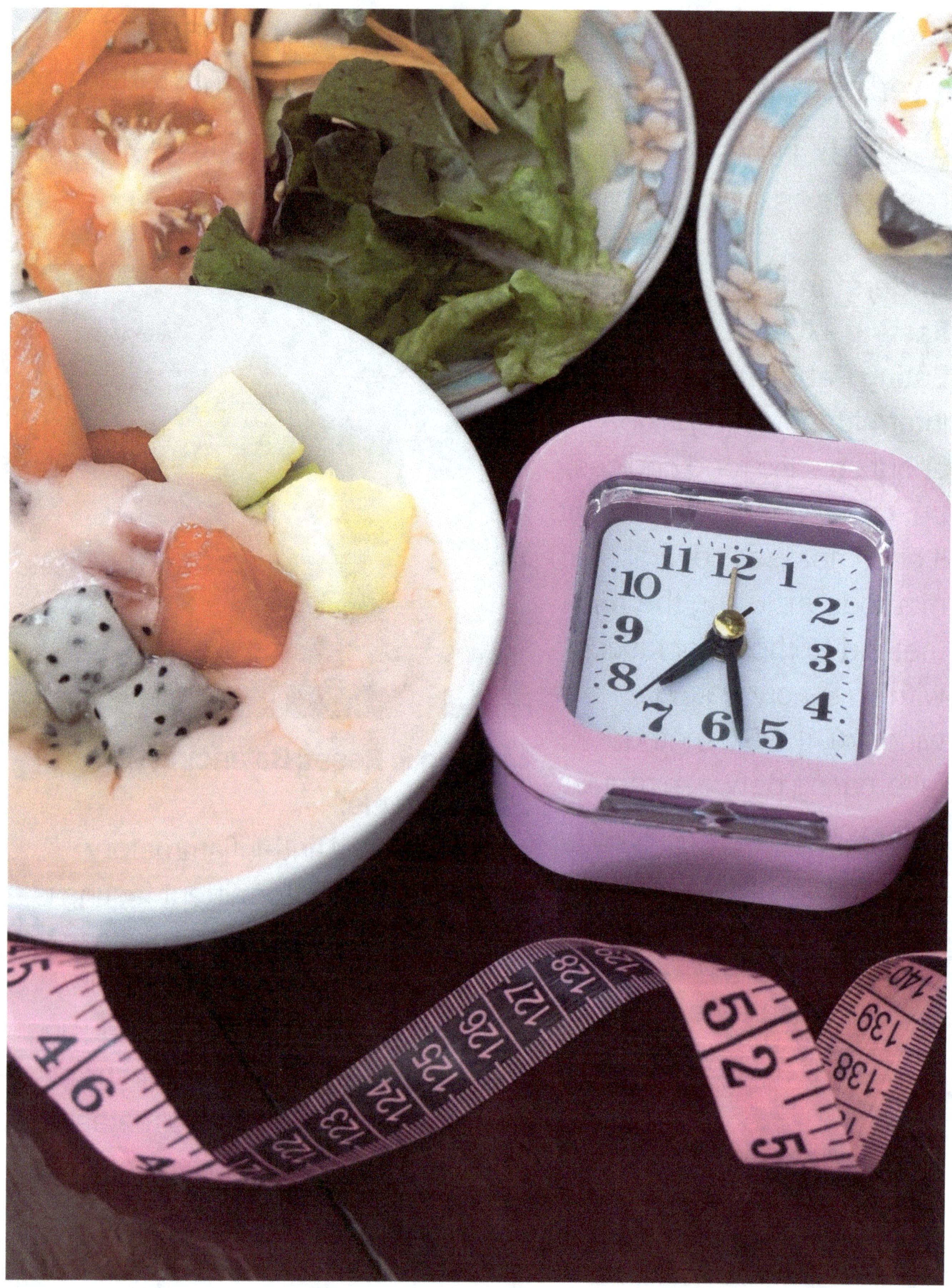

Autophagy: Cellular Cleansing for Inflammation Management: Intermittent fasting induces a cellular process known as autophagy, in which the body removes damaged cells and cellular components. This self-cleansing mechanism not only promotes cellular health, but also reduces inflammation by eliminating sources of oxidative stress and dysfunctional cellular elements.

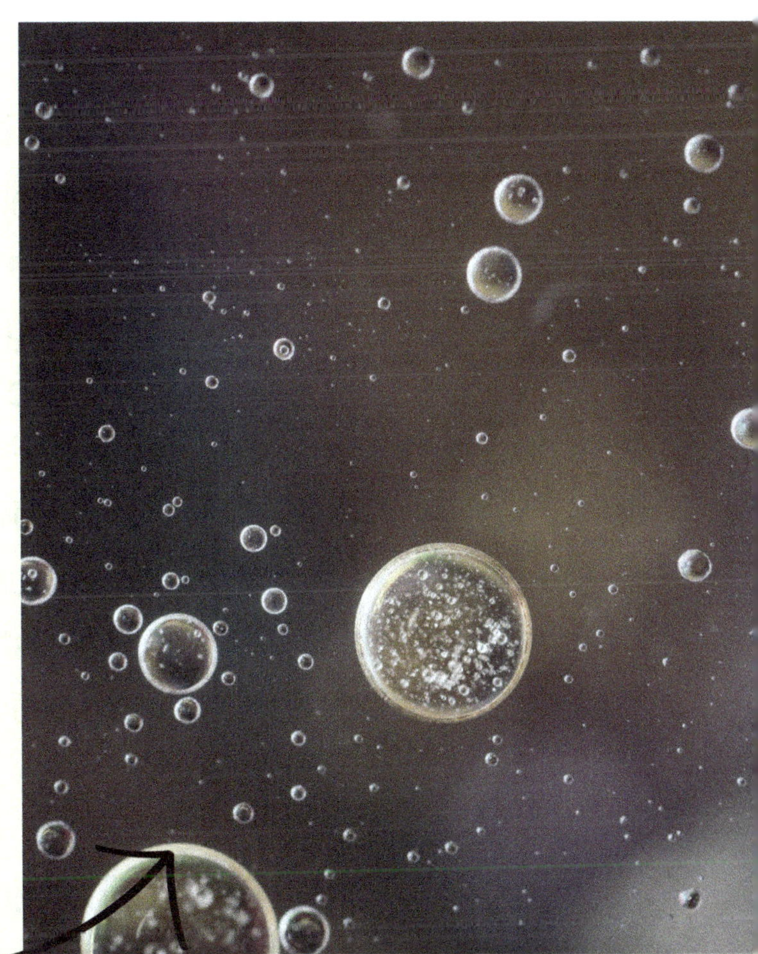

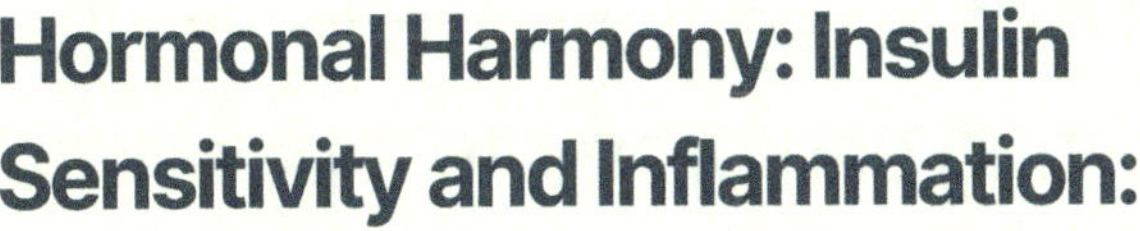

Hormonal Harmony: Insulin Sensitivity and Inflammation: Intermittent fasting increases insulin sensitivity, which improves the body's ability to regulate blood sugar. This in turn reduces the risk of chronic inflammation, as insulin resistance is closely linked to inflammatory processes. By promoting hormonal balance, intermittent fasting contributes to an anti-inflammatory internal environment.

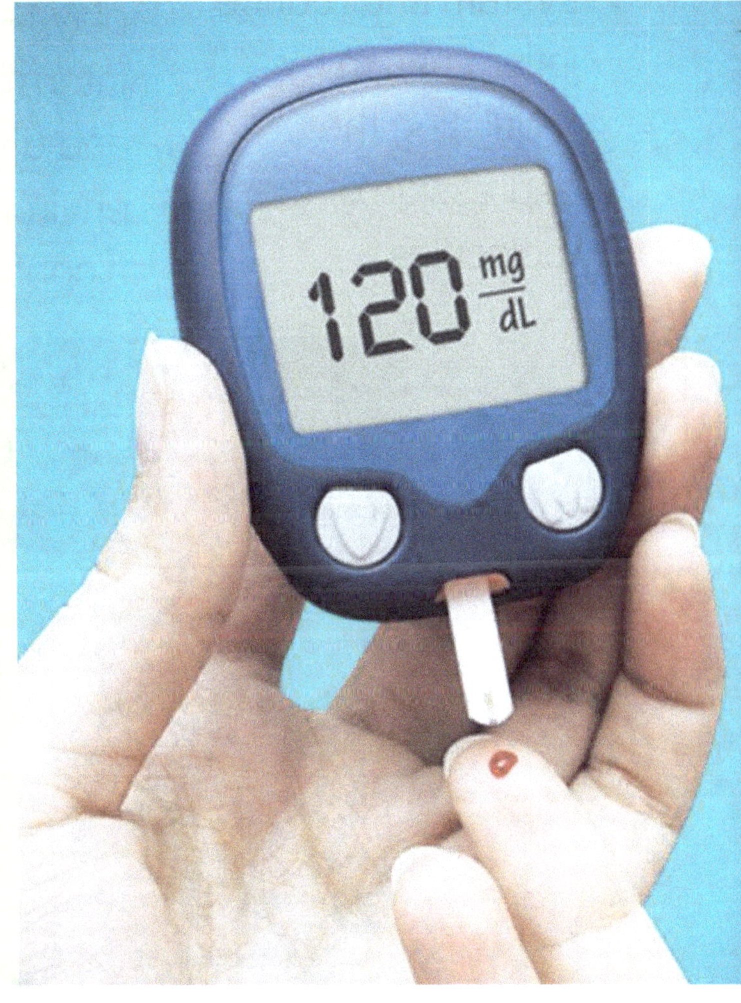

Modulating Cytokines

Studies suggest that intermittent fasting may affect the production of pro-inflammatory cytokines, which are signaling molecules that play a role in the inflammatory response. Intermittent fasting helps to balance the immune system and reduce inflammation by regulating the expression of these molecules.

Oxidative Stress Reduction

Intermittent fasting regimens help reduce oxidative stress by incorporating periods of fasting. Oxidative stress, which results from an imbalance between free radicals and antioxidants, is a major contributor to inflammation. By acting as a proactive measure, intermittent fasting helps guard against inflammatory damage caused by oxidative stress.

Gut Microbiome

The gut microbiome is a community of microorganisms in the digestive tract that plays a crucial role in regulating inflammation. Intermittent fasting can promote a balanced and diverse gut microbiome, creating an environment that supports overall health and a controlled inflammatory response.

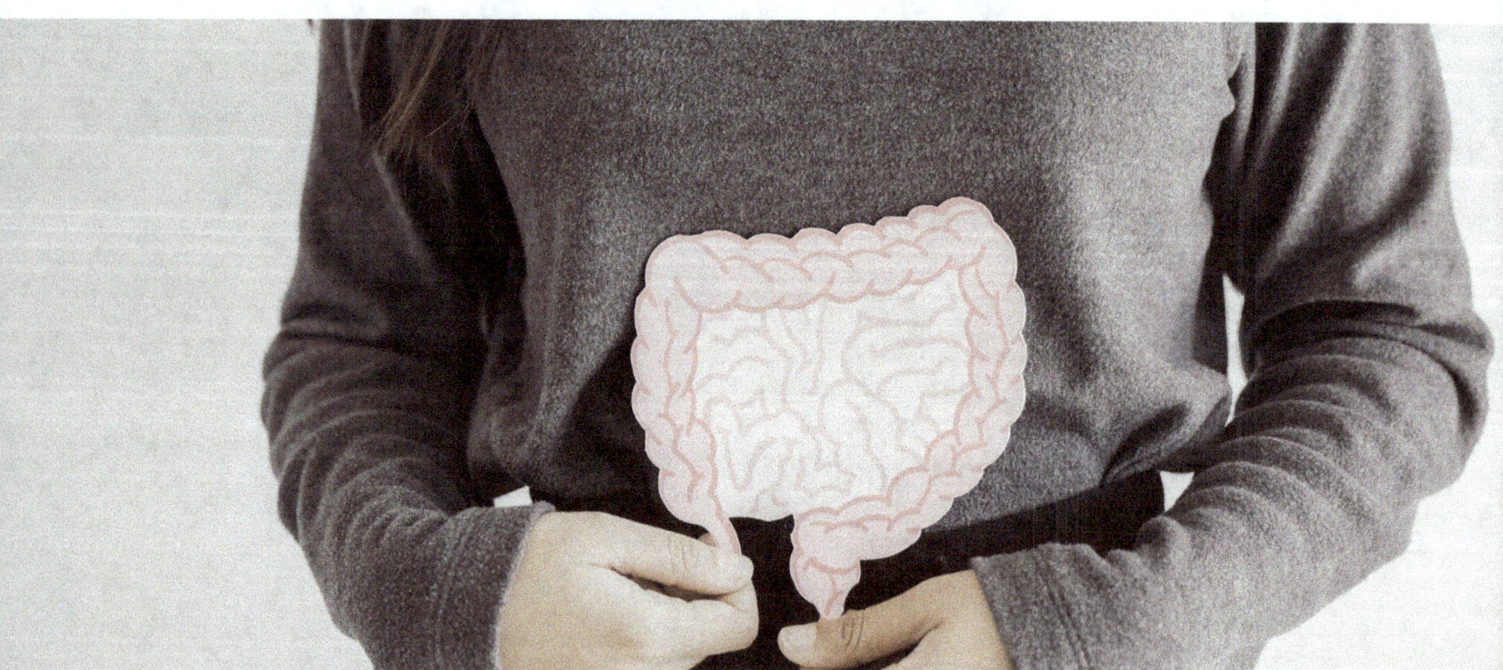

Personalization and Adherence — Intermittent fasting's effectiveness varies among individuals. Personalization and adherence are key to success. Experiment with different fasting methods and find a schedule that aligns with your lifestyle and preferences for long-term sustainability.

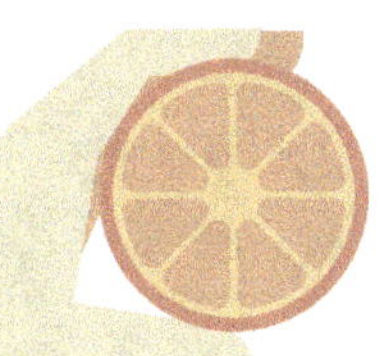

Navigating Intermittent Fasting Safely — Before starting intermittent fasting, consult a healthcare professional, especially if you have pre-existing health conditions. To minimize potential side effects, make gradual adjustments to fasting periods and practice moderation.

Hydration and Nutrient Intake — Proper hydration and nutrient intake are crucial for overall health during intermittent fasting. Staying hydrated aids in the detoxification process, while nutrient-dense meals enhance the body's anti-inflammatory capacity.

Although intermittent fasting has anti-inflammatory benefits, it should be viewed as part of a holistic wellness strategy. To achieve optimal health and vitality, it is important to combine intermittent fasting with a nutrient-rich diet, regular physical activity, and stress management.

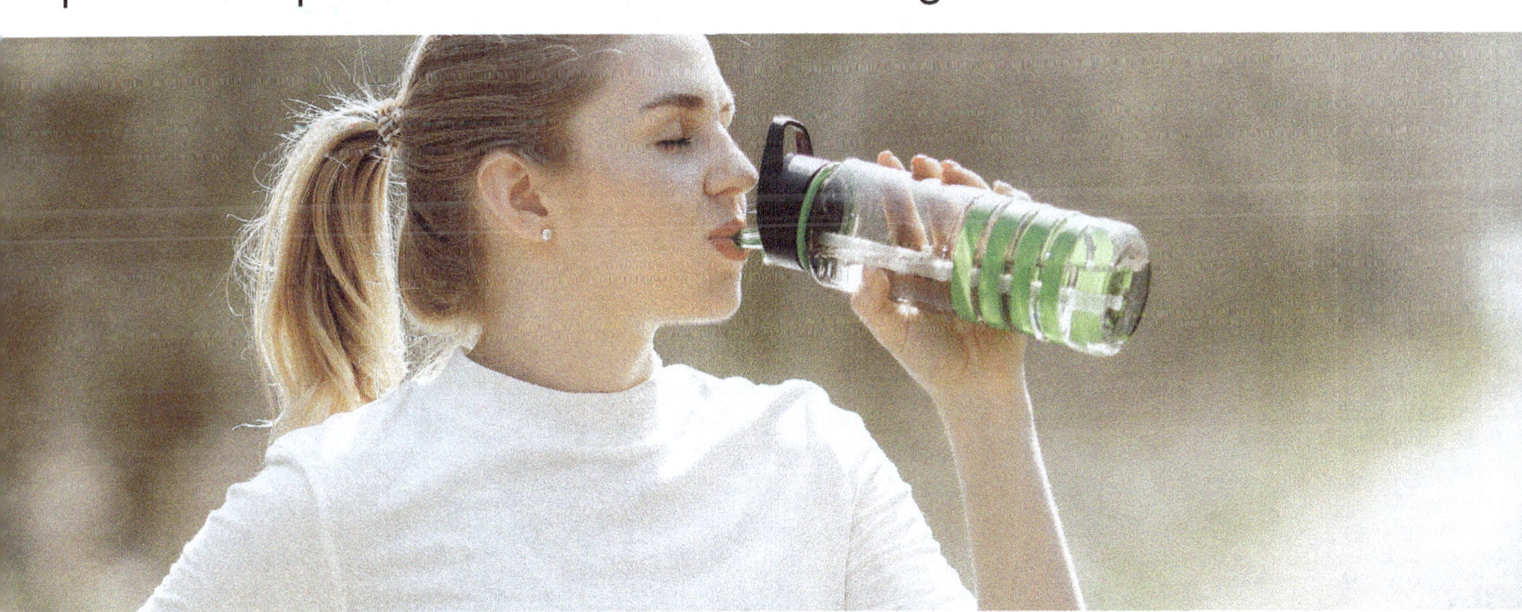

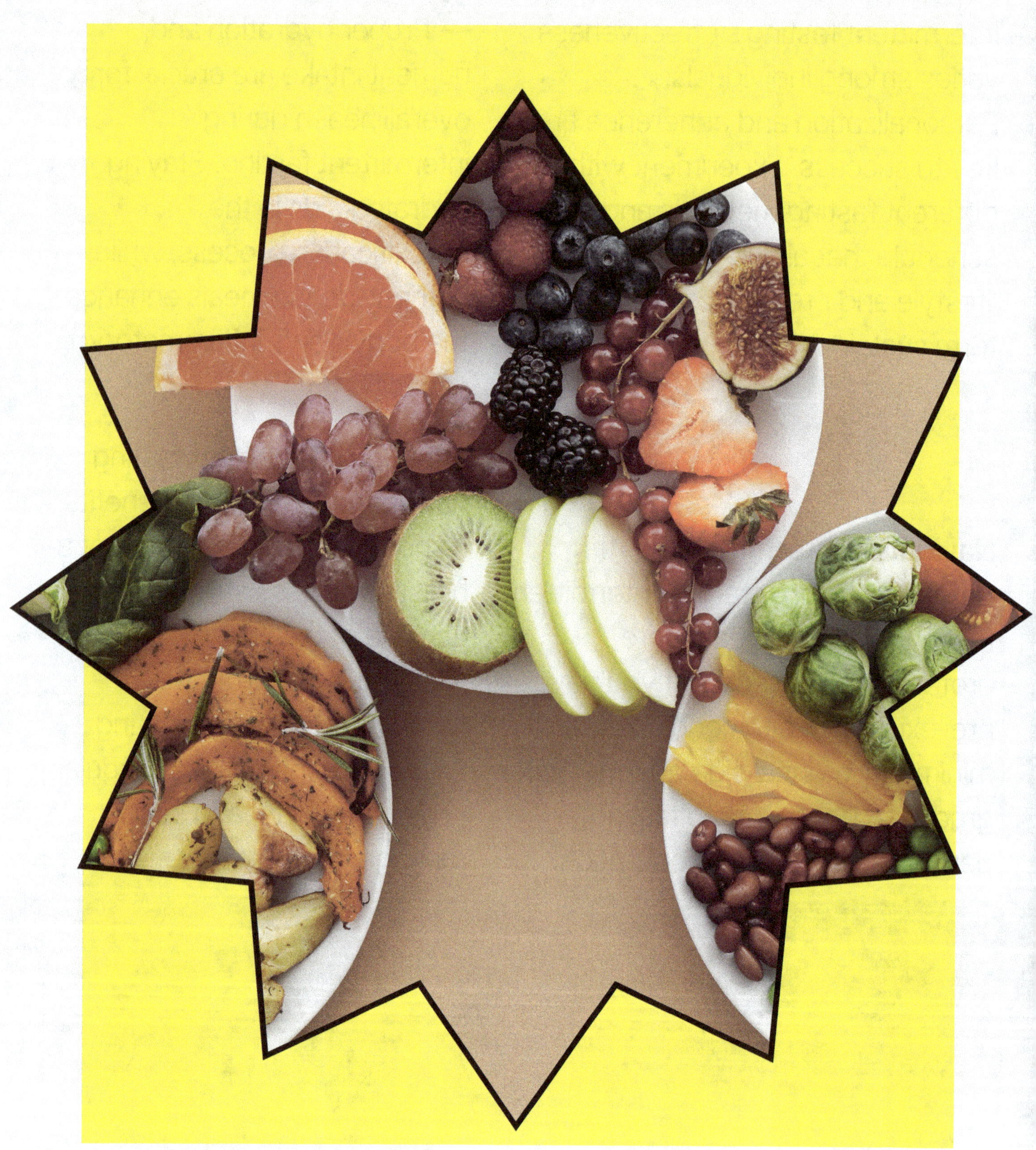

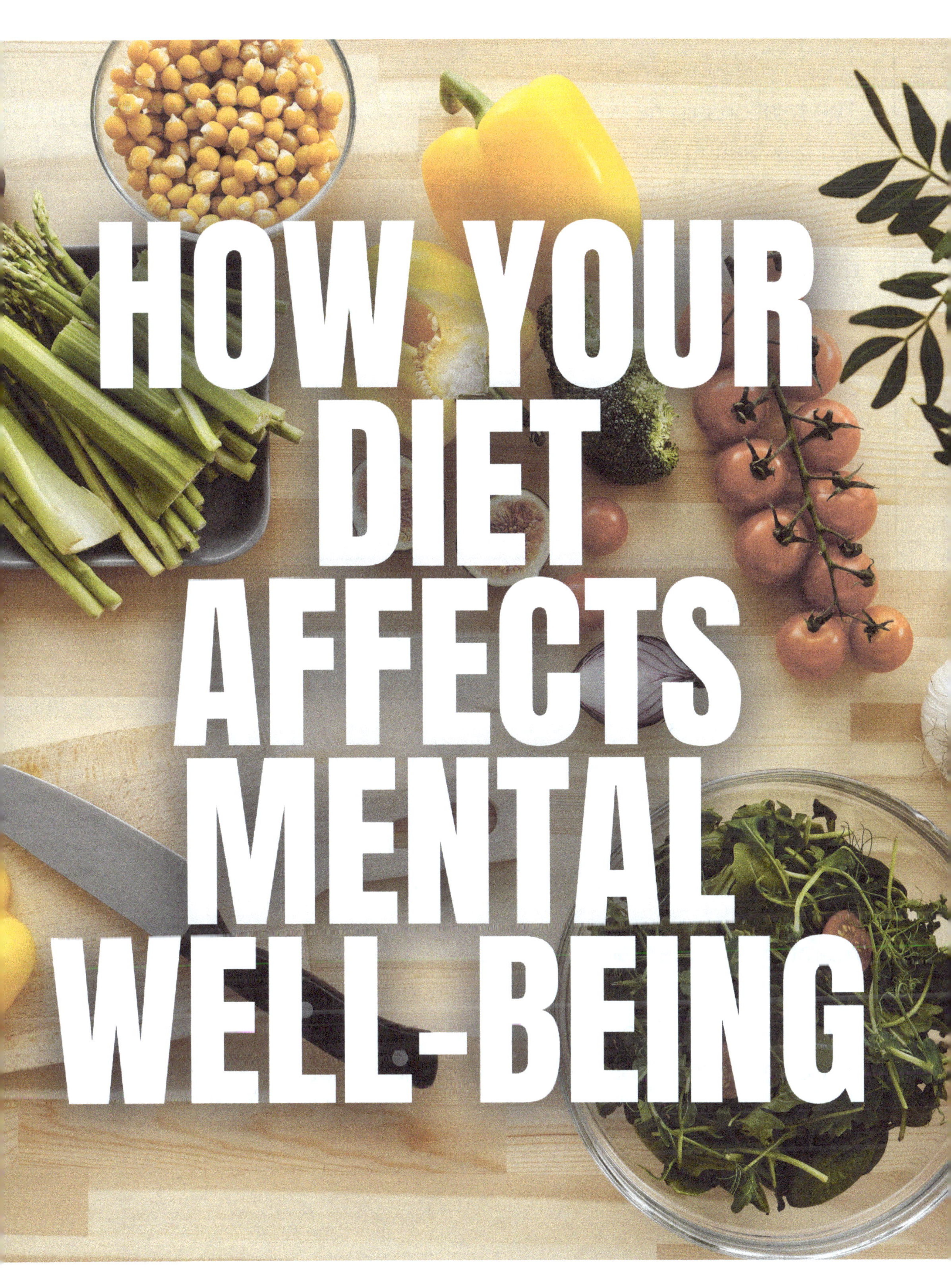

HOW YOUR DIET AFFECTS MENTAL WELL-BEING

The relationship between the gut and the brain is a fascinating and pivotal axis that profoundly influences our physical health and mental well-being. The gut-brain connection involves a dynamic interplay of signals and interactions. The food we consume serves as a potent communicator between these two vital command centers. The gut-brain connection is a scientific topic that we will explore. Our mental health can be significantly impacted by the choices we make in our diets.

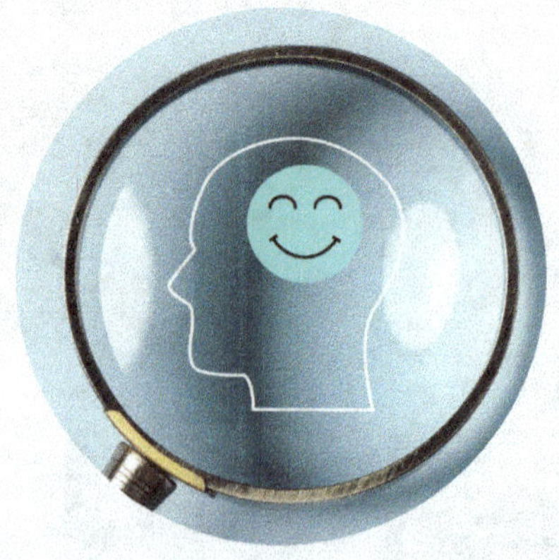

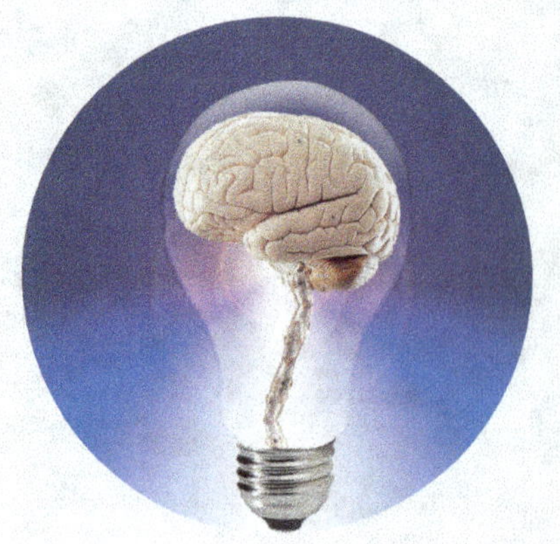

The "Second Brain" in Your Gut —
The gut has a complex network of neurons called the enteric nervous system (ENS), also known as the 'second brain.' This network is embedded in the walls of the digestive tract and communicates with the central nervous system (CNS). It plays a crucial role in regulating digestion and influencing emotional well-being.

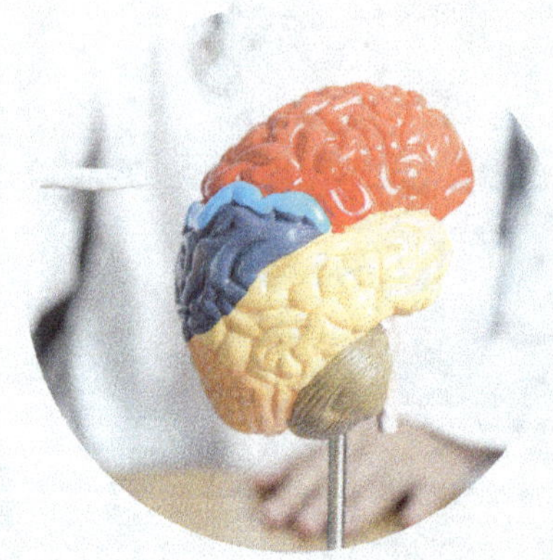

Probiotics and Mental Resilience — Probiotics, beneficial bacteria, can have a positive impact on mental health. They contribute to a balanced microbiome, which fosters an environment that supports mental resilience and may even help reduce symptoms of anxiety and depression.

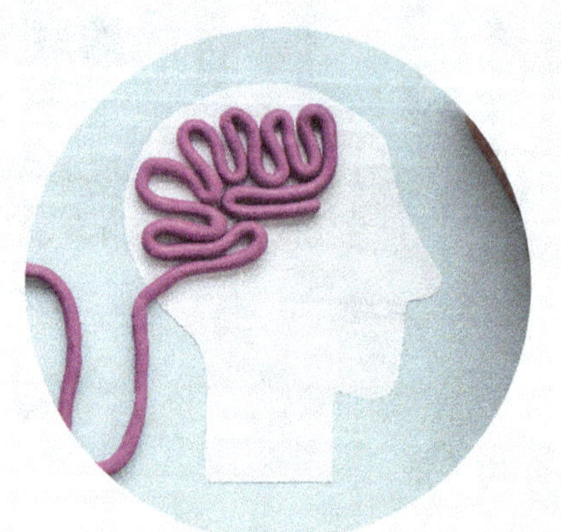

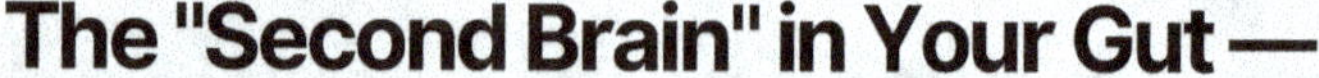

Short-Chain Fatty Acids — During the fermentation of dietary fibers, the microbiota produces short-chain fatty acids (SCFAs), including butyrate. These SCFAs have been linked to anti-inflammatory and neuroprotective effects, and play a crucial role in maintaining a harmonious gut-brain relationship.

Fueling Brain Functionality — The nutrients from our food are crucial for brain function. Absorption of nutrients in the gut directly affects cognitive processes, memory, and overall mental acuity. A diet rich in vitamins, minerals, and antioxidants supports optimal brain health and contributes to mental well-being.

The connection between the gut and the brain is closely linked to the inflammatory response. A diet that is high in processed foods, sugars, and unhealthy fats can cause inflammation in the gut, which may lead to inflammation in the brain. Mental health conditions such as depression and anxiety are associated with chronic inflammation.

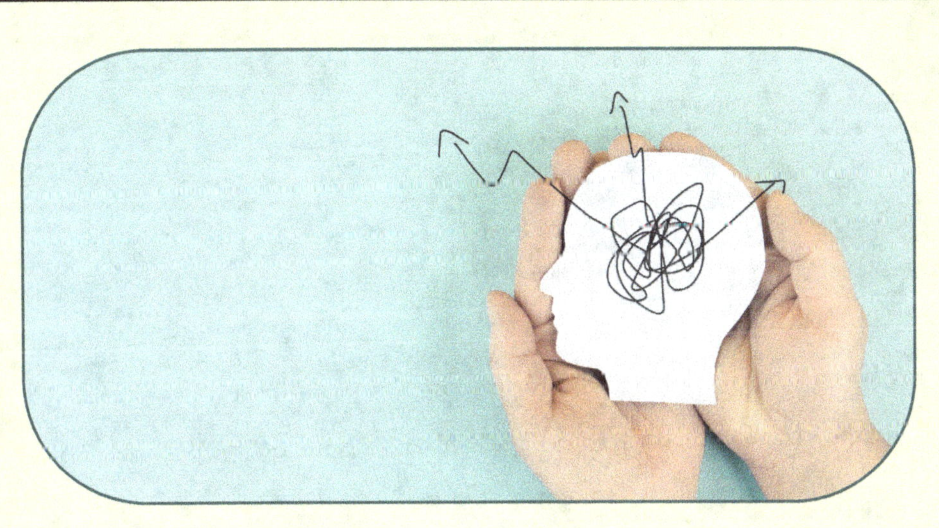

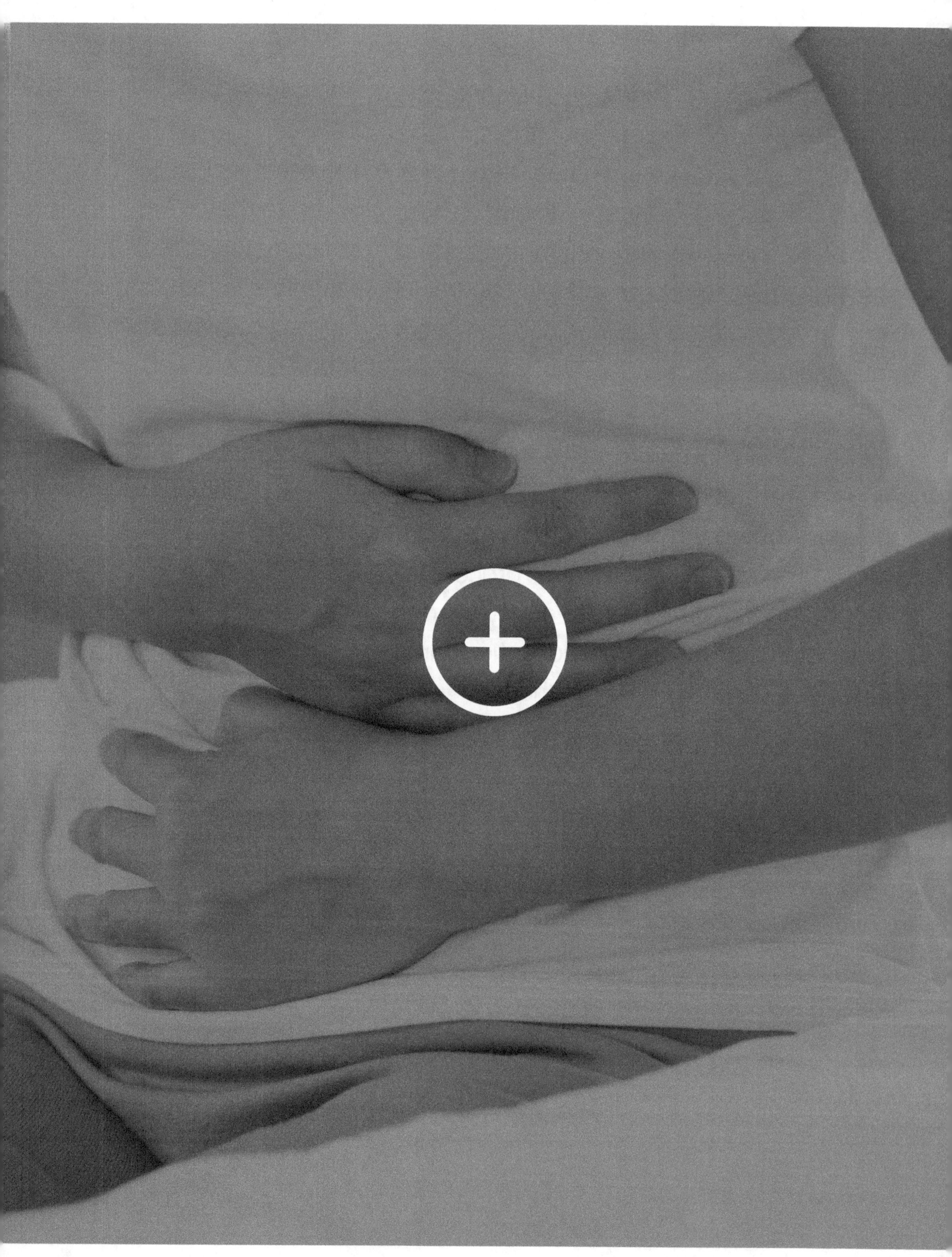

Navigating the complex gut-brain connection requires us to make thoughtful and mindful choices in our diets. **These choices have an impact beyond digestion, nurturing our mental well-being and fostering a harmonious interplay between the gut and the brain.** Embracing a diet that supports a diverse microbiome, reduces inflammation, and prioritizes nutrient-rich foods can lead to a symphony of nourishment. This symphony resonates not only in our physical health but also in the profound landscape of our mental and emotional vitality.

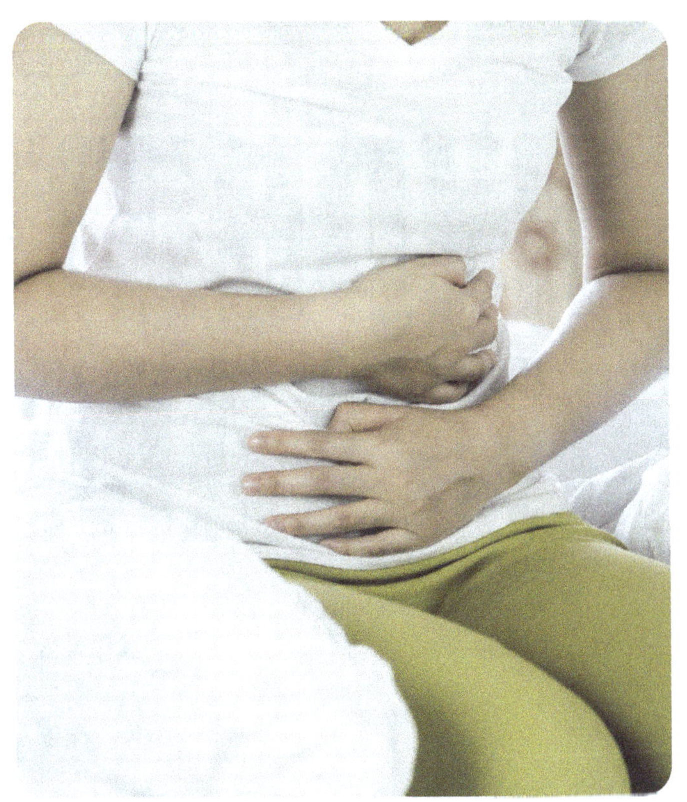

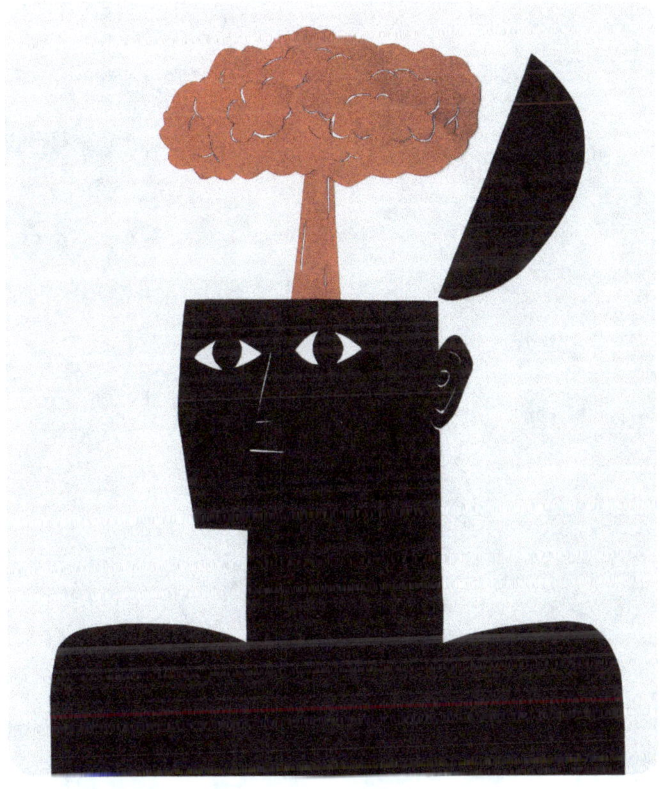

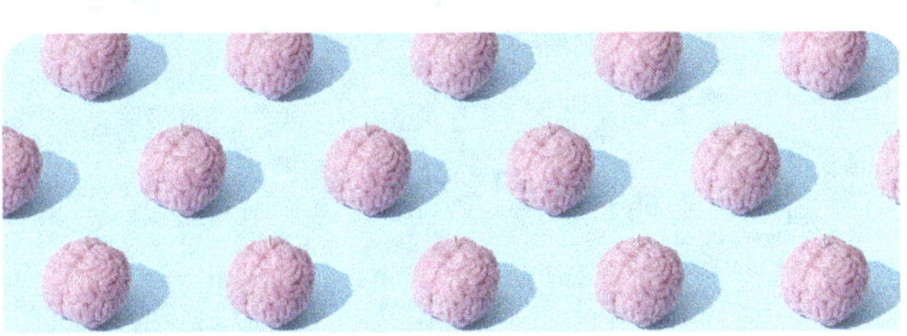

HYDRATION AND INFLAMMATION

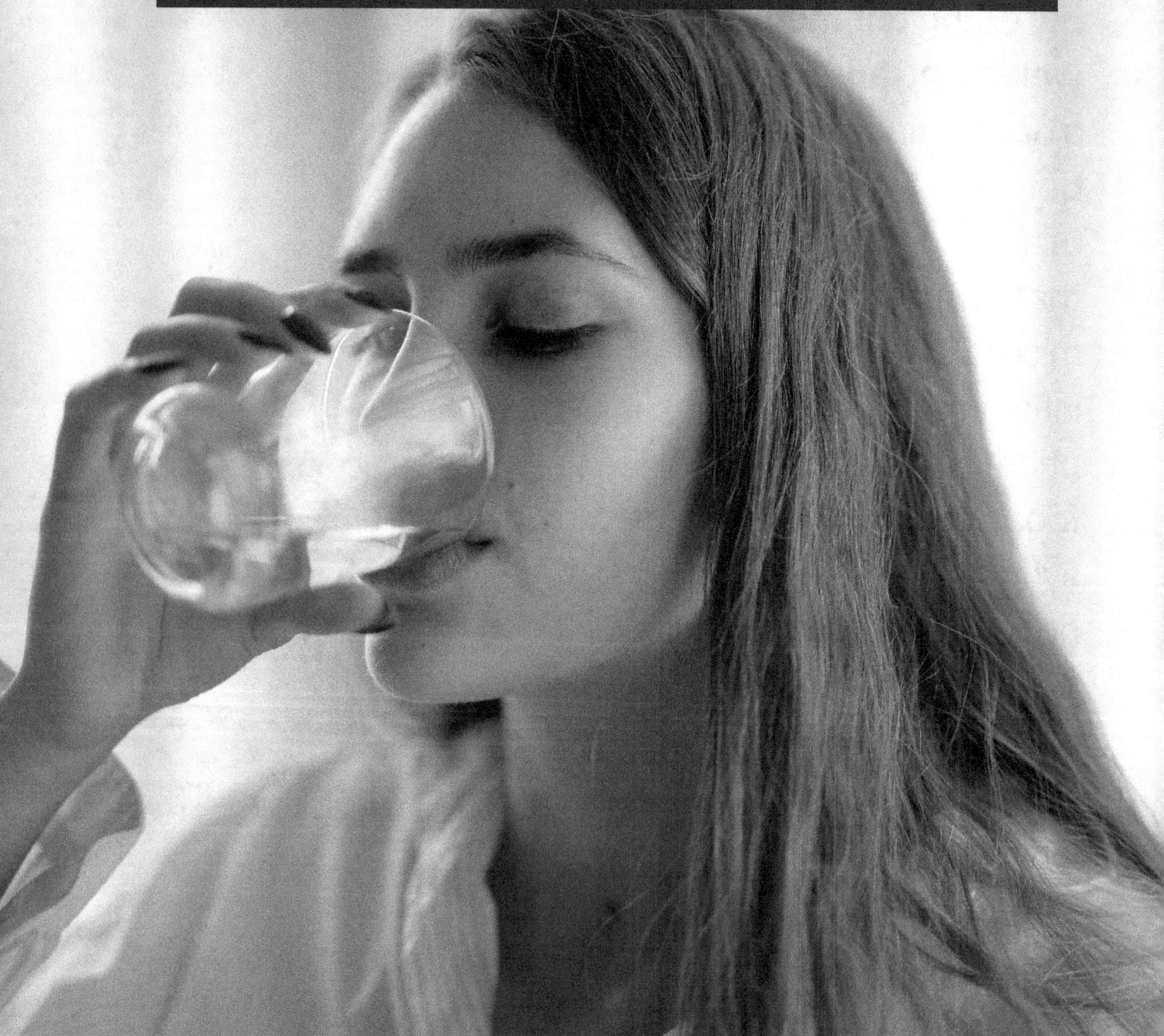

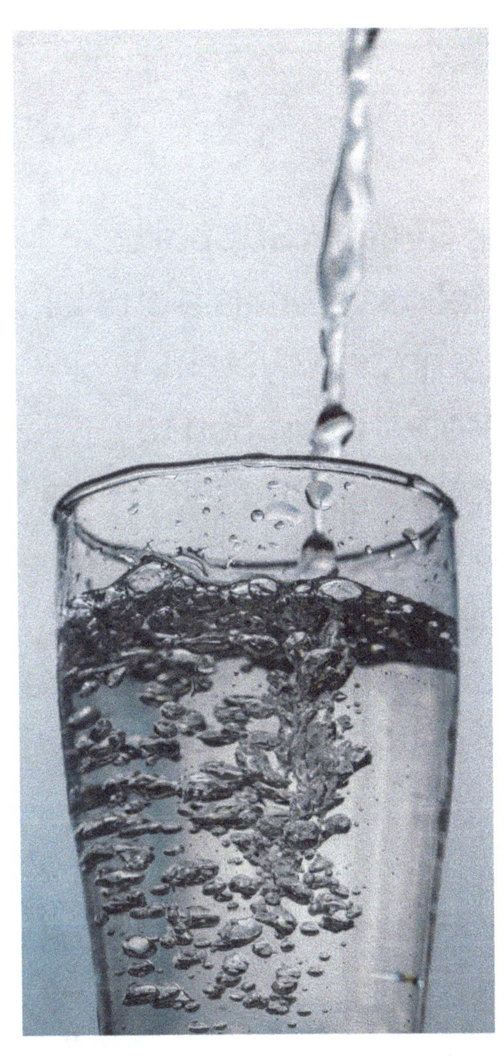

Hydration is essential for our body's functionality. It is not just about quenching thirst, but a fundamental physiological need that affects every aspect of our body. Water is vital for nutrient transport, temperature regulation, and waste elimination.

Water as a Solvent -
Proper hydration is crucial for transporting nutrients throughout the body. It acts as a solvent, helping essential nutrients reach cells and tissues. Adequate nutrient delivery supports the body's ability to regulate inflammation and maintain optimal function.

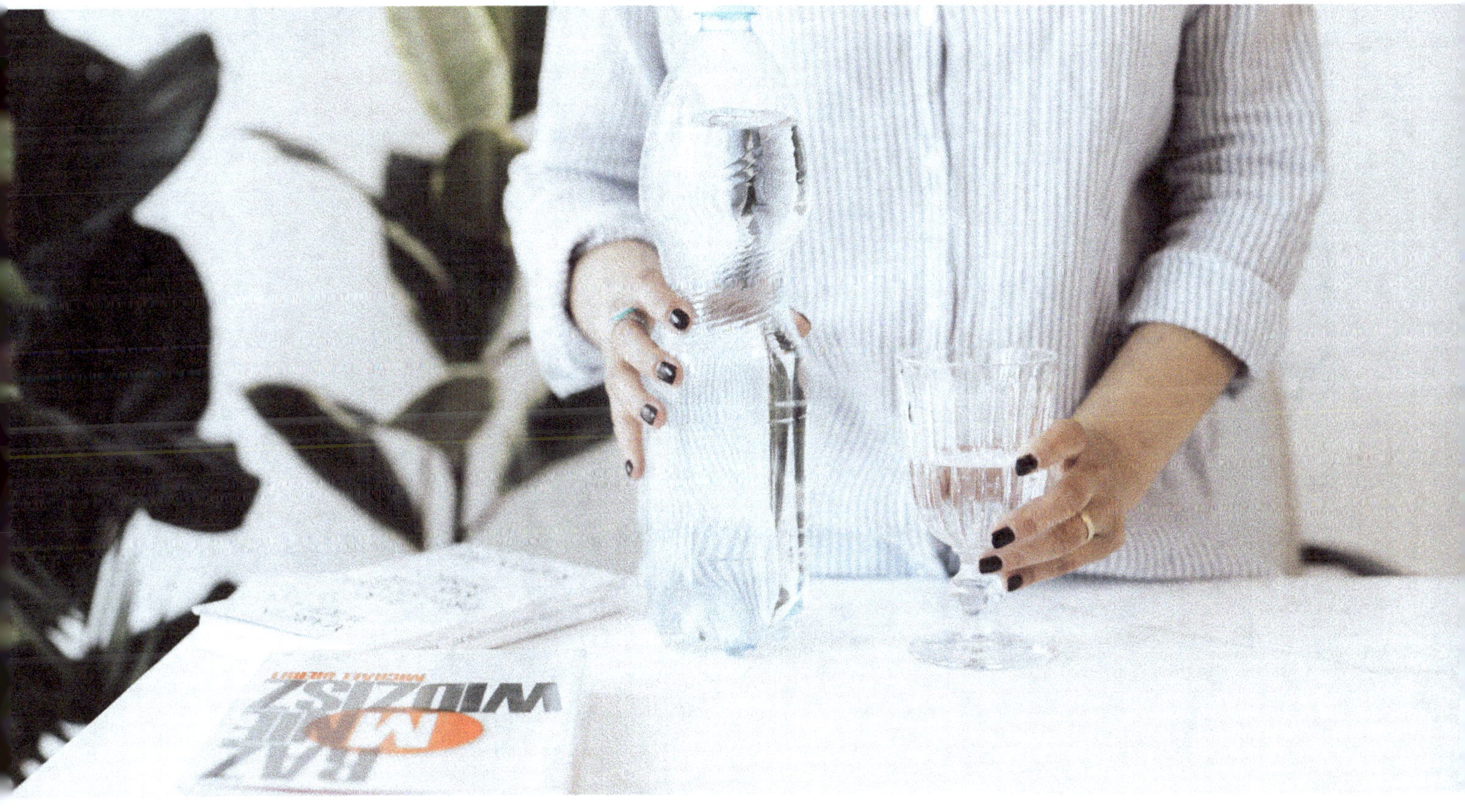

1

A Guardian Against Inflammatory Imbalance

Maintaining fluid balance is crucial for the body's homeostasis. Dehydration disrupts this delicate equilibrium, leading to a concentration of inflammatory mediators in the blood. Staying adequately hydrated helps the body manage inflammation and reduces the risk of chronic inflammatory conditions.

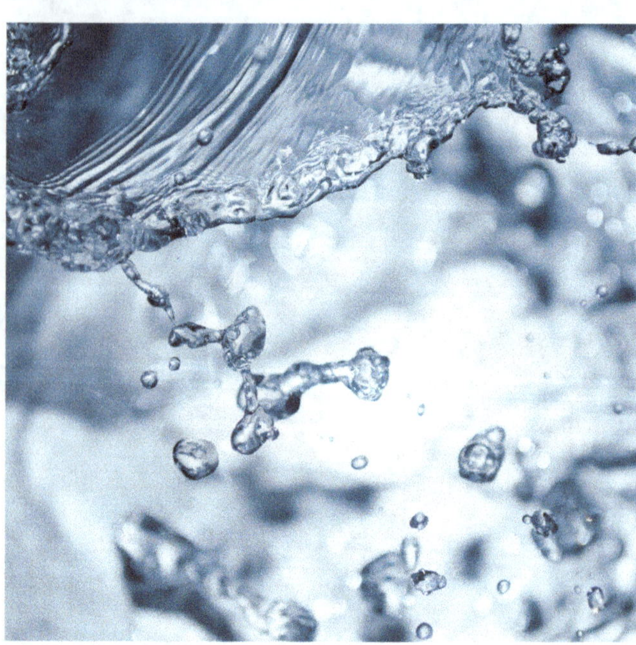

2

Lymphatic System Support

The lymphatic system is a crucial part of the immune system. It relies on proper hydration to function optimally. Adequate fluid levels help the lymphatic system clear toxins, waste products, and inflammatory substances from the body. This contributes to a balanced and healthy immune response.

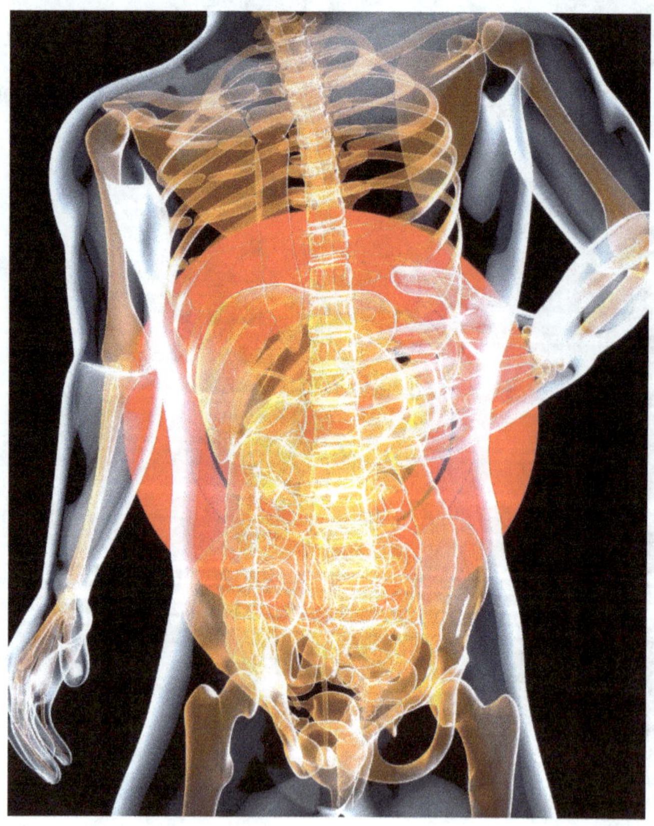

KIDNEY FUNCTION

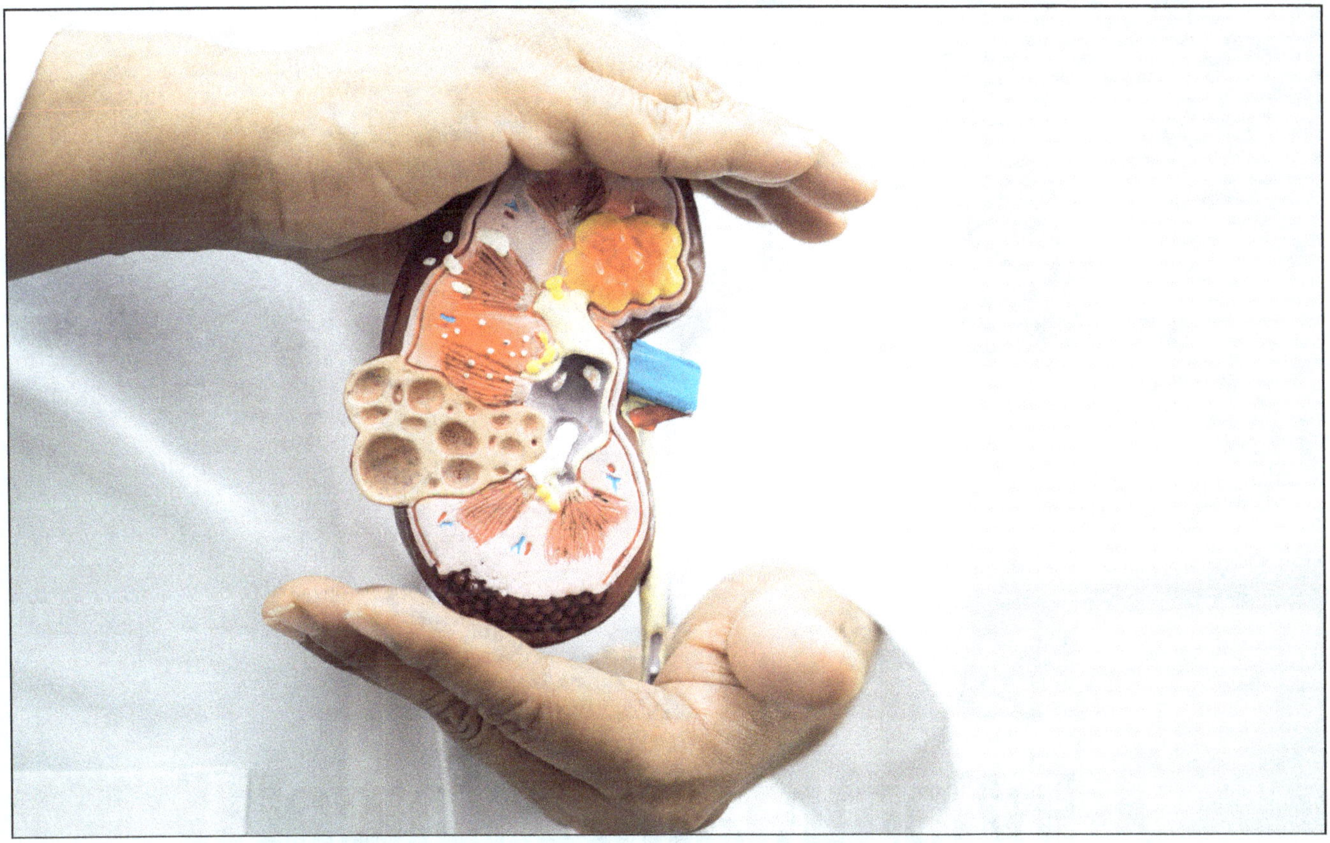

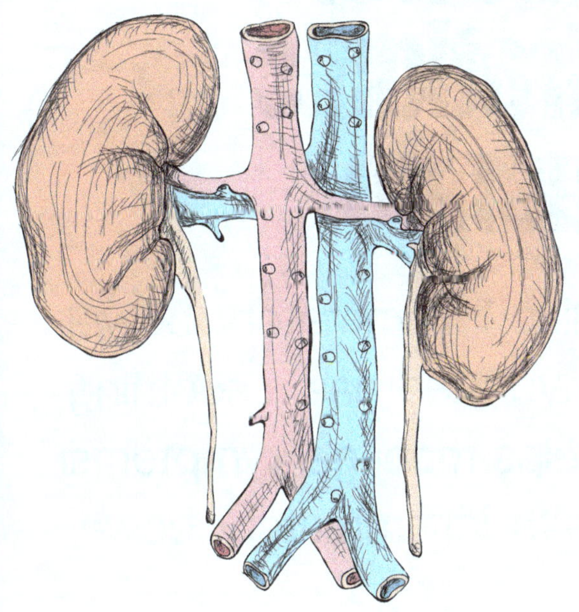

Filtering Out Inflammatory Triggers

The kidneys filter waste products and inflammatory substances from the blood. Optimal kidney function is supported by proper hydration, which ensures efficient toxin removal and maintains a balanced internal environment that discourages inflammation.

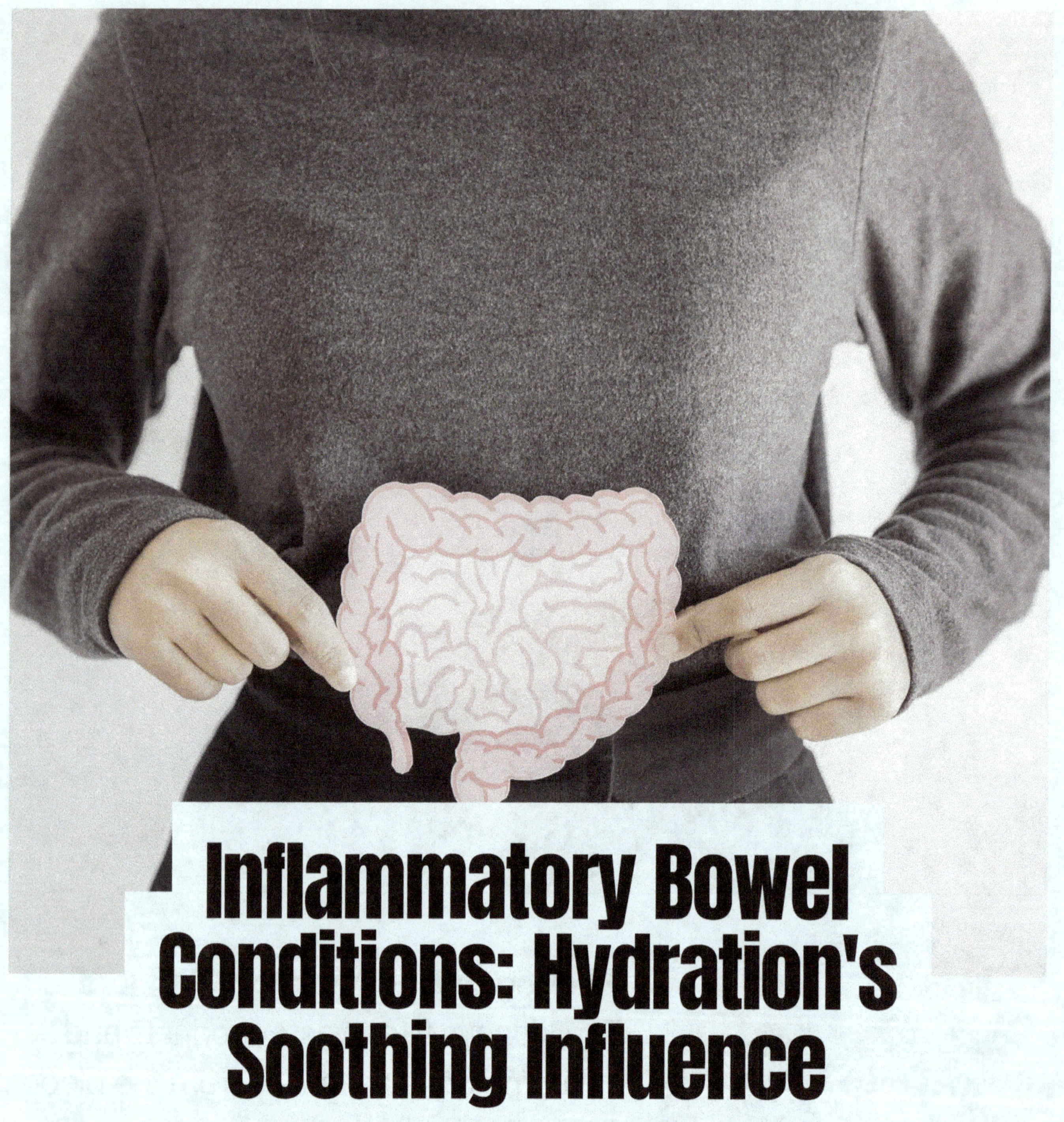

Inflammatory Bowel Conditions: Hydration's Soothing Influence

Dehydration can worsen conditions like inflammatory bowel disease (IBD). Keeping yourself well-hydrated has a soothing effect on the digestive tract, which helps manage symptoms and reduce inflammation in people with inflammatory bowel conditions.

It plays a vital role in balancing the body and should not be underestimated. Ensure the text is grammatically correct, uses simple vocabulary, and is accessible to a broad audience. Avoid adding new content or changing the meaning of the original text. Hydration is a crucial element in managing inflammation and maintaining overall well-being. Keep sentences short and straightforward, use active voice, and present information in a logical order. Use verb phrases instead of noun phrases and aim for standard, simple sentence structure. Recognizing water as the overlooked elixir empowers us to sip wellness, extinguishing the inflammatory fire within and fostering a state of internal balance that resonates with vitality and health.

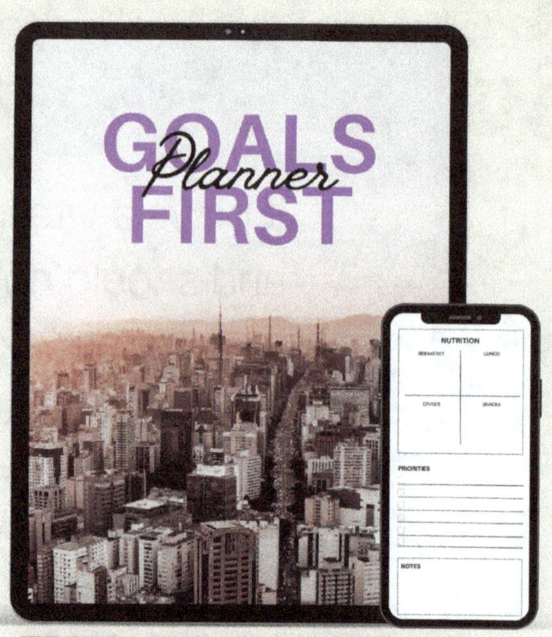

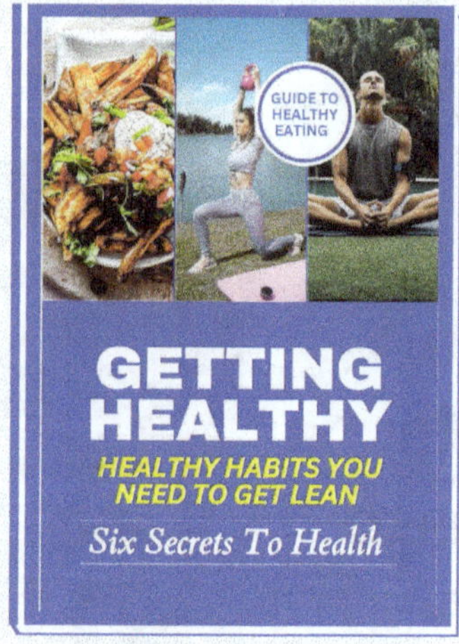

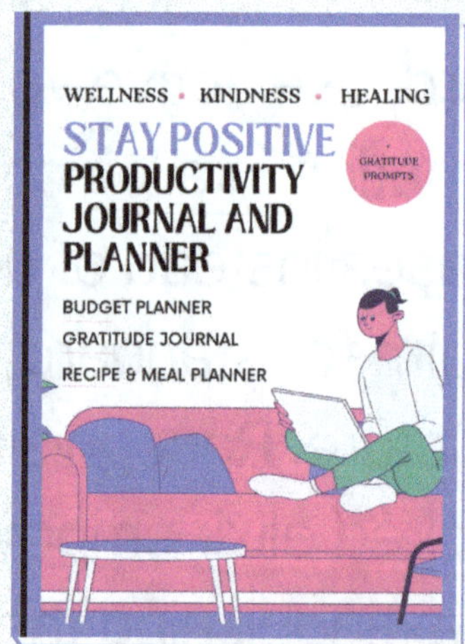

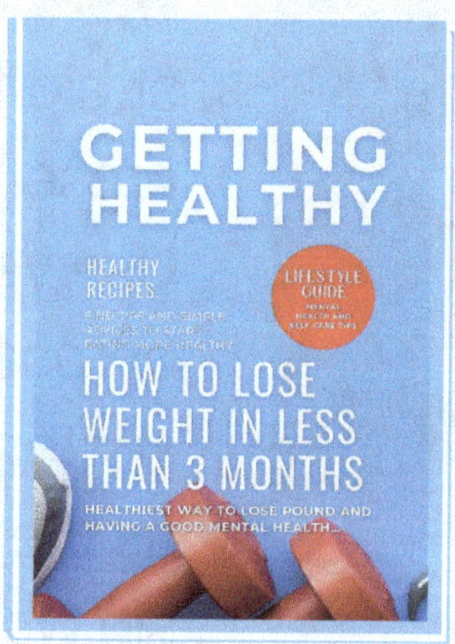

The Ultimate Guide To Living a Healthy Lifestyle: How To Improve Your Life with Food, Exercise and Self–Care

A Gratitude Journal and Planner for Personal Growth with Journaling Prompts

A Practical Guide for Achieving Optimal Health, Shedding Pounds, and Cultivating Lasting Habits

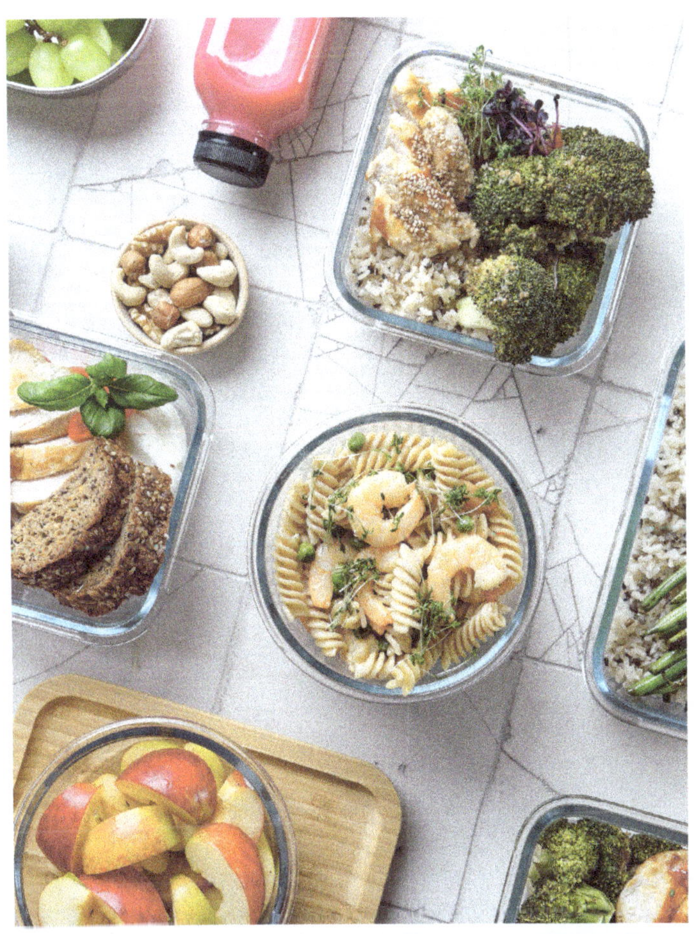
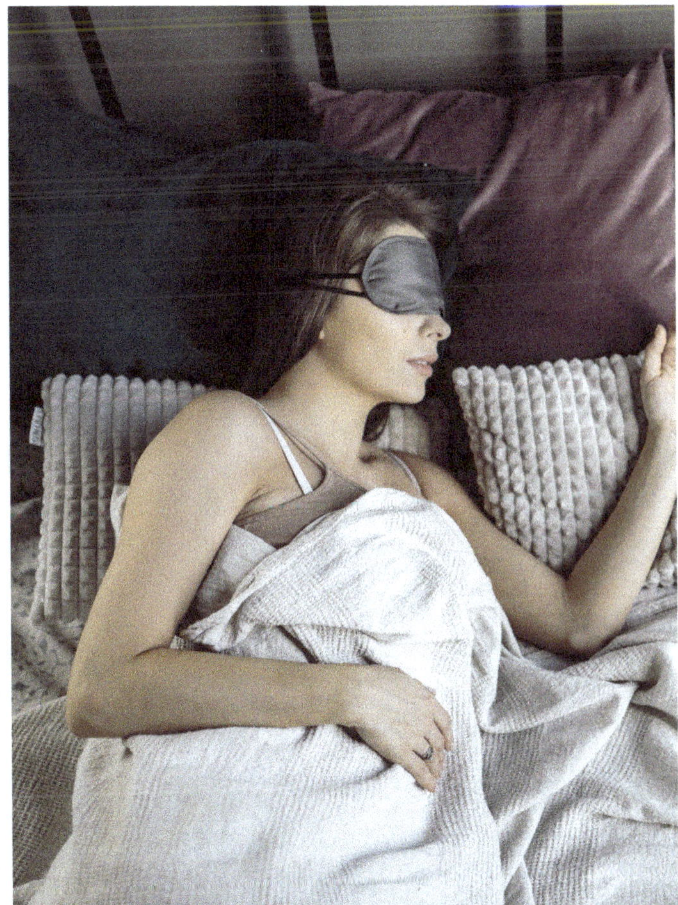
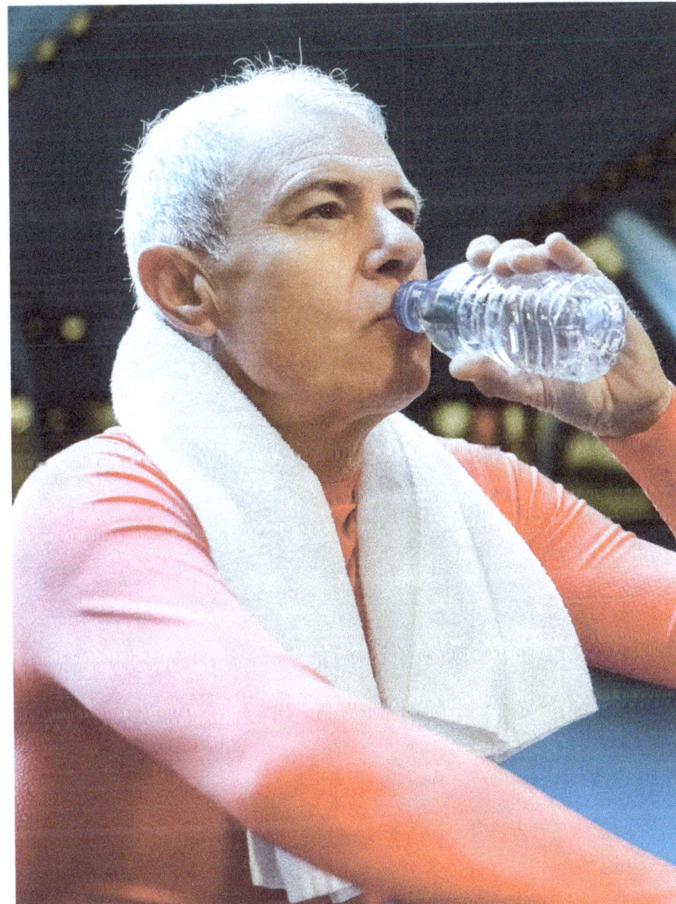
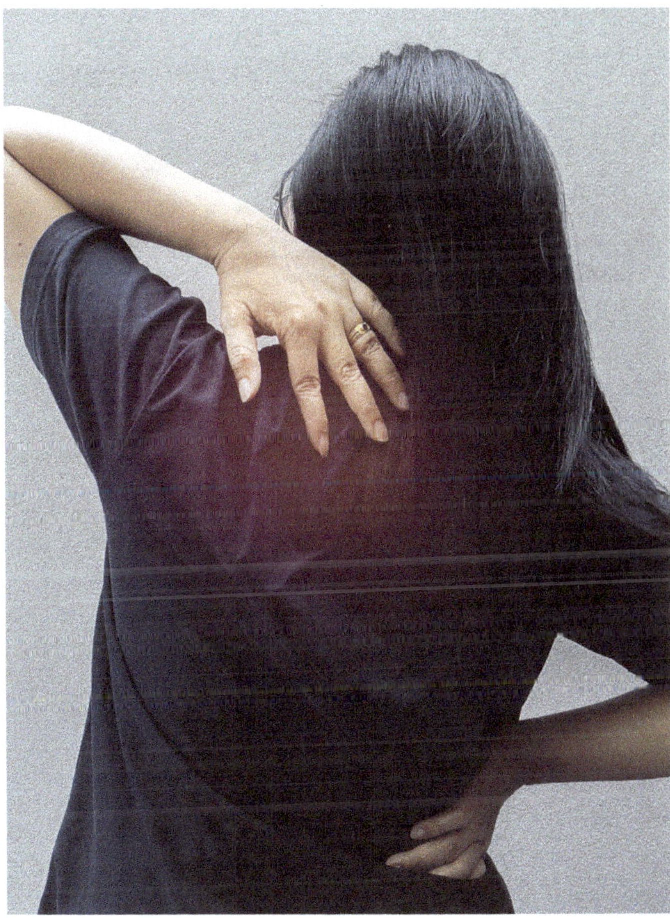